Diagnosis of Gastrointestinal Parasitism in Dogs and Cats

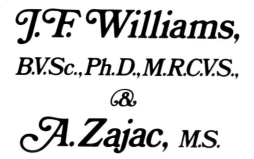

J.F. Williams,
B.V.Sc.,Ph.D.,M.R.C.V.S.,
&
A.Zajac, M.S.

Department of Microbiology and Public Health
College of Veterinary Medicine
Michigan State University
East Lansing, MI 48824

Introduction

There has been a remarkable increase in the number of dogs and cats per household in the USA in recent years (Nowell, 1978). Consequently, veterinarians are being called upon with greater frequency to provide professional services and judgment in the treatment, management and control of diseases of these pets. Problems caused by gastrointestinal helminths and protozoa have become especially important because of the changes which have occurred in our understanding of their biology and significance as causes of disease in animals and in man. These factors make it timely to review and illustrate the diagnosis of parasitism in companion animals. With this in mind, we have assembled a series of photographs of diagnostic features of the principal parasites found in the dog and cat. They are presented here together with our comments on the interpretation of laboratory tests, and on the need for careful consideration of the history, clinical findings and epidemiology in arriving at conclusions and recommendations.

In the past, diagnosis of parasitic infection has been based all too often upon the relatively simple criterion of the presence or absence of eggs, larvae or cysts in the feces of infected animals. Some quantitative estimate of the intensity of infection was then generally arrived at through a scoring procedure related to the number of eggs, *etc.*, per sample or unit of sample. While the laboratory detection and identification of parasitic stages in feces is still a fundamental part of diagnosis, clinical experience and research findings in a variety of experimental models have made it clear that many factors can influence the success of these tests. For example, female parasites do not produce eggs constantly, and under the influence of host immunity, diet, host physiologic status, or even the season of the year, egg or larva production may be inhibited partially or completely for long periods. As a result, even when large and pathogenic worm burdens are present, they may not always be detectable. We have also come to recognize recently that severe clinical disease can occur in the prepatent period, *i.e.*, when eggs, larvae or cysts are not shed because no fertile mature parasites have yet developed. This is especially important in the light of the remarkable efficiency of perinatal transmission mechanisms. Through either intra-uterine migration or by transfer in colostrum or milk, many parasites can accumulate in the intestines of suckling puppies or kittens. Their pathogenic effects may be fatal even before eggs or larvae appear in the feces.

The necessity for accuracy in diagnosis is underscored by the increasing public awareness of the potential for human infection by parasites of dogs and cats.

Recognizable syndromes of visceral larva migrans, cutaneous larva migrans, zoonotic strongyloidosis and toxoplasmosis have now been well defined in children. These diseases, coupled with the occasional and unusual instances of accidental parasitism (*e.g.* by *Dipylidium* tapeworms), have given rise to serious concern about the role of companion animals as hazards to human health. When this awareness in the pet-owning public is combined with the unfamiliarity of physicians with parasitic organisms, the potential for unreasonable and unnecessary antagonism towards pets is created. This can be effectively countered by the adoption of sound positions by veterinary practitioners, based upon their comprehension of the biology and transmission of the agents involved, and the reliability of the diagnostic procedures which they use. Adding further to the responsibility of the veterinarian in this area is the increasing tendency of owners and their families to travel with pets, even overseas. Parasites which were formerly exotic or restricted to certain regions in the USA have now become factors to consider in the diagnosis of parasitism in small animal practice in all parts of the country.

The situation in which veterinary practitioners are placed, both in relation to the health of their patients and their clients, is made all the more difficult by the dearth of adequate research on specific questions involving parasitism in dogs and cats. Thus the zoonotic implications of *Giardia* infections of young puppies and kittens are unclear. The relationship between intestinal helminthiasis and the syndrome of eosinophilic enteritis is not resolved. The relevance of recent findings on relationships between gastrointestinal parasites of cattle and pathophysiologic disturbances in secretion, absorption and motility of the gut, and on the hormonal status, and growth and performance of the host, is frustratingly difficult to assess in terms of comparable helminth infections in dogs and cats. Veterinarians often, then, find themselves unable to take advantage of these developments in trying to apply modern medicine in small animal practice.

We obviously have much to learn in determining the importance of parasites as agents of disease in dogs and cats, rather than simply responding to their presence when detected through the microscope. The need for further research to address these questions is evident, and is clearly linked to the diagnostic problems which they pose. In some instances in the review we have taken the opportunity to point up some of the important deficiencies which must be considered by investigators in the future.

II

Table of Contents

        Dipylidium
        Taenia
        Echinococcus
        Hymenolepis
        Mesocestoides
        Diphyllobothrium
        Spirometra

        Physaloptera
        Toxocara
        Toxascaris
        Trichuris
        Ancylostoma
        Capillaria
        Strongyloides
        Filaroides
        Aelurostrongylus
        Angiostrongylus
        Spirocerca

        Alaria
        Paragonimus
        Fasciola
        Nanophyetes
        Amphimerus

RALSTON PURINA COMPANY: Checkerboard Square, Saint Louis, Missouri 63188

© Copyright 1980 by Ralston Purina Company.
Copyright under the International Copyright Union.
All rights reserved.
This book is protected by copyright.
Made in the United States of America.

Photographs reproduced by permission.

Library of Congress catalog card number: 80-80293
First printing, 1980

Sample Collection for Diagnosis of Parasitism

In the vast majority of cases, the diagnosis of gastrointestinal parasitism involves the processing of fecal samples. A variety of techniques has been developed by which to examine these and in the following section we have detailed some reliable procedures, though these are by no means to be considered necessarily better than standard methods in reference texts. However, some important points regarding sample collection should first be made because they can influence the success of laboratory diagnosis and often do not receive proper emphasis.

It is always best to obtain fresh fecal samples. Failing that, one should at least learn something about the age and source of the sample. Many parasitic organisms undergo quite rapid developmental changes soon after they are voided in feces, and their new forms may become very difficult to recognize. Hookworm eggs, for example, in warm humid weather hatch very rapidly giving rise in 24 hours or so to active, motile larvae in old fecal samples. On the other hand, the presence of motile larvae in fresh feces has an altogether different significance, and requires consideration of lungworm infection or strongyloidosis. Similarly, *Toxascaris* eggs become embryonated within a few days in old feces in the environment, but they are normally passed unembryonated in fresh samples. In contrast, the presence of embryonated smooth-shelled eggs in fresh feces points to nematodes such as *Physaloptera*. At

the other end of the scale, certain parasites deteriorate very rapidly after being passed in the stool, so that samples which are not fresh are useless for the detection of motile *Trichomonas* or *Balantidium* trophozoites.

By insisting on collection of fresh samples, the reliability of identification of source is also increased. Left to their own devices, clients may scrape old feces from the lawn or litter. These may or may not have come from the patient in question. Fecal samples when passed on soil quickly become invaded by a variety of organisms such as free-living nematodes, larvae of flies and other arthropods. Their presence may then lead to misdiagnosis or controversy, often resolved only by collection and processing of yet another sample. When clients witness the passage of samples which are collected fresh, they are also less likely to submit specimens of vomitus in place of feces, since in some disorders they may be readily confused. In addition, it provides an opportunity for the owner to make useful observations on the form of the fresh sample. The presence or absence of blood-tinged mucus, for example, may be diagnostically significant, *e.g.*, in *Trichuris* infections, but very difficult to detect in samples which are old. Freshly-passed samples may bear visible segments of tapeworms on their surface but these are very active and may leave the stool and in a matter of hours the sample may prove negative. Also, if the feces are exposed to the environment for any length of time, tapeworm segments may become dried or disintegrated and difficult to recognize. Insects and birds find motile tapeworm segments attractive and sometimes will devour them before they can be detected in the laboratory.

Desiccation is generally harmful to parasites and care must always be taken to avoid drying. The sample, once collected, should be kept refrigerated in order to avoid further development of parasite embryos or zygotes. A small plastic or waxed cardboard cup with a snap-on lid makes a useful container. Samples should weigh at least two grams (about equivalent to one teaspoonful). If dogs are hospitalized, feces may be obtained from the rectum. In fact, the collection of fresh rectal samples is preferable for diagnosis of infection with labile protozoa, or *Strongyloides* larvae which may be more numerous on the rectal wall.

If the sample is to be preserved, it should be placed in a larger container and thoroughly mixed with enough 10% formalin (see Appendix) to produce a loose, soupy mixture; too little formalin or inadequate mixing will not preserve parasites. Unfortunately, formalin fixation can lead to distortion of protozoan trophozoites and cysts and, of course, will kill motile parasitic larvae. Fresh material must be tested if these types of infections are suspected. It is also worth pointing out that fixation with formalin will not usually inhibit further development of Ascarid ova, nor will it reduce the infectivity of eggs of *Toxocara* or *Echinococcus*. This is particularly important in view of the public health importance of these parasites.

Once again, the characteristics of the stool sample on arrival ought to be noted by the veterinarian or technician before laboratory tests are done. Gross visual inspection of feces is especially valuable in cases of tapeworm infection where individual ova may not be present in the fecal mass and where the diagnosis is going to depend on observing the presence of mature proglottids. It is at this time that abnormal color, consistency or odor can be recorded, along with comments on the presence or absence of mucus or blood. Careful observation can be helpful in detection of bright red blood which might indicate *Trichuris*, or the dark, tarry color of blood lost in the small intestine as a consequence of hookworm infection.

Laboratory Diagnostic Procedures

The most common procedure for the detection of internal parasitic infection is based on the concentration of ova, larvae or cysts by selective flotation. In many small animal practices this technique is used exclusively. For several reasons, however, we recommend that routine processing of fecal specimens should include the use of both the direct smear and flotation techniques.

The importance of the direct examination of feces is often overlooked by veterinarians and technicians. Although the fecal flotation test is very successful in the diagnosis of most common parasitic infections, a number of parasites are destroyed or unrecognizably damaged by the hypertonic flotation solutions. Protozoan organisms are particularly susceptible to the effects of saturated sugar and salt solutions and the presence of amebae or *Trichomonas* may be entirely overlooked unless a direct smear is made of the feces. Similarly, helminth larvae, like those of *Strongyloides*, unprotected by tough eggshells, may be distorted almost beyond recognition by dense flotation solutions.

The direct fecal examination is also useful in detecting parasite ova which are too dense to float consistently in the kinds of saturated sugar solutions often used in flotation tests. On the other hand, sedimentation procedures for detection of ova are cumbersome and are rarely performed in most practices. Consequently, exclusive use of flotation tests might well preclude detection of certain fluke infections and limits the rate of detection of the more dense ova of worms such as *Spirocerca* and *Physaloptera*.

DIRECT SMEARS

In performing a direct examination of feces a small amount of material should be collected on the end of a wooden applicator stick and mixed with a drop of water or saline on a microscope slide. The edge of the cover slip can be used to push larger pieces of material to the side and the remainder of the fluid is then covered and examined. If protozoan organisms are suspected but difficult to demonstrate, a drop of Lugol's parasitological iodine (see Appendix) may be added to the fecal smear.

One difficulty in making direct smears is that they often are not made thin enough to read easily, and if the feces contain a high proportion of coarse particles, even experienced practitioners may have difficulty evaluating slides. A further and more significant disadvantage of the direct exam is that only a very small portion of the fecal sample is being tested. Like the flotation test, the direct exam should never be used alone in the diagnosis of internal parasitism. Instead, it should be an important complement to the flotation test as part of the routine examination of feces. Even in the busiest practice, the direct exam will provide enough valuable information to justify the few extra minutes needed to perform it.

FECAL FLOTATION TEST

The basis of the fecal flotation test is that parasite ova and cysts can be separated from other similarly sized fecal debris because of differences in density. The products of parasitic infections (eggs, oocysts, larvae) are usually less dense than flotation solutions, and therefore will rise to the surface of the mixture where they can be collected and examined. Obviously, this allows one to examine a larger and more representative sample of the feces.

A number of readily available compounds can be used to produce saturated solutions effective in the flotation tests, including sucrose, sodium chloride, magnesium sulfate, and zinc sulfate (see Appendix). Saturated sucrose, although historically the most commonly used solution, is less dense than saturated solutions of salts, and will not permit flotation of all fluke and nematode ova. In addition, the high viscosity and stickiness of the sugar solution increases the difficulty of handling and of maintaining a clean lab area. Saturated salt solutions are more convenient as flotation media; however some variation in efficacy amongst these solutions occurs. We have found that the most consistent results are obtained with anhydrous zinc sulfate. Unfortunately, the higher density of zinc sulfate, which results in flotation of almost all fluke and nematode eggs, also causes collapse of some ova. When zinc sulfate is used, slides should be examined with this consideration in mind.

Several variations in the technique of the fecal flotation exam are described in the literature, but the following is one which we have found to be reliable in the regular processing of fecal material:

1. Approximately one to two grams of feces are combined and mixed thoroughly with about 10 ml of flotation solution, with care being taken to avoid too much bubble formation.

2. This mixture is strained through cheesecloth into a 15 ml centrifuge tube and more flotation solution is added until a convex meniscus is visible at the top of the tube.

3. A coverslip is then placed on the meniscus at the top of the tube which is centrifuged for approximately three minutes at 1500 rpm (if no centrifuge is available, the tube should be left undisturbed on the bench for at least 30 and preferably 60 minutes).

4. Following centrifugation the coverslip is removed from the top of the tube, placed on a microscope slide and examined under the scanning objective (5-10x) of a compound microscope. If the slide has to be kept beyond the time required for immediate inspection, petroleum jelly or a mixture of approximately ⅔ petroleum jelly and ⅓ mineral oil should be placed in a thin layer along the edges of the coverslip. This is conveniently done by smearing a small amount of the jelly on the palm or a finger and dragging each edge of the coverslip through it in turn until the perimeter is completely rimmed. Slides prepared in this way can be kept for several weeks if refrigerated at 4°C in a moist environment. A covered petri dish containing moistened paper towelling serves this purpose well.

MICROSCOPIC EXAMINATION

An initial water wash of the feces may be performed to remove fine particulate material and produce a cleaner slide for examination. Feces are mixed with water, filtered through cheesecloth and centrifuged for 5 minutes at 1000 rpm. The supernatant is then discarded and the sediment mixed with flotation solution, taking care to disperse clumps of material evenly into the solution. Steps 2-4 of the basic flotation test can then be carried out. In instances where the construction of the centrifuge does not allow use of glass coverslips, the tube need not be completely filled with flotation solution. After centrifugation, the parasite ova may be removed by lightly touching the surface of the fluid with the flattened end of a glass rod or wooden applicator stick. This material is then deposited in a drop of water or saline on a microscope slide, cover slipped and examined. Currently, there are several commercial fecal flotation exam kits available which contain the necessary materials for the test and do not require the use of a centrifuge. Generally, slides prepared with these kits can be read 10-20 minutes after combination of feces with the flotation solution.

Two points need to be emphasized in the examination of slides by either the direct or flotation exam. Firstly, scanning of the slide must be performed in an inclusive and consistent manner, either from top to bottom, or side to side. Where egg or cyst numbers are low, haphazard examination of the slide simply cannot be depended upon to detect infections. Scanning of slides is most effective if the objective lens is no greater than 10x. Higher power lenses should only be used for detailed examination and identification of material located with the lower power. All too often inexperienced operators try to scan with high power lenses. This is tedious and inefficient and leads to inaccuracy. The second point is that slight alterations of the plane of focus as the slide is scanned are invaluable in identifying ova or cysts. Diagnostic characteristics of parasite materials may only be detected if there are changes in focus as the slide is scanned and the use of the fine adjustment is a great aid. In addition, one may find that the plane of focus shifts markedly if the coverslip is not perfectly horizontal. When this happens eggs or cysts may not be seen unless the fine adjustment is in constant use.

Experience is probably the most important factor in the consistent discrimination of parasite material from other fecal constituents, although some general guidelines may be helpful. On the whole, artifacts or pseudoparasites of plant or fungal origin do not show the constancy of form and size characteristic of parasite ova and cysts. This will become apparent as the whole coverslip area is examined. Likewise, the frequency with which one encounters the structure can be a useful indicator, since many artifacts may be sporadic or rare. If this is borne in mind, the presence of one unusual structure with some resemblance to a known parasite egg can be quickly discounted as insignificant. Diagnosis of a parasitic

infection based on a single confusing or questionable specimen on the slide should not be attempted. If there is some uncertainty, an additional fecal sample should be collected and examined.

In cases where parasite larvae are present, detection is generally easier, but it should be remembered that free-living nematodes are common soil inhabitants, and they will quickly invade fecal material once deposited on the ground. As a rule, these free-living nematodes are larger and contain more complex internal systems than parasitic larvae. In particular, the presence of eggs in the uteri of female worms clearly distinguishes soil nematodes from parasite larvae. Free-living mite ova and insect larvae should also be recognized as artifacts. The presence of typical farm animal parasite eggs or oocysts in the sample will result from coprophagy or accidental ingestion of ruminant, hog or horse feces. Rodent or bird parasite ova often appear in the feces of cats and dogs which hunt. If pseudoparasitism is suspected, control of the diet or hospitalization for several days is necessary before repeat sampling.

An appreciation of the organisms making up the normal parasitic fauna of the host animals is helpful in making decisions about some of these materials, and the illustrations we have assembled in the following sections should serve to identify the most common agents. Even more critical in the successful identification of parasitic infections is the awareness of the relative sizes of ova and cysts. Knowledge of the absolute measurements of the organisms may be useful, but it is not essential if one has reliable standards of comparison for determining size. These standards may relate parasitic ova and cysts to one another and to common types of fecal debris, and development of this awareness of size is an essential skill in the accurate and reliable identification of parasitic infections. We have included a scale bar in all of the photographs. The relative sizes can best be gauged by reference to the figures in Chapter 5 in which all of the diagnostic forms are shown as seen at the same microscopic magnification.

SEDIMENTATION

Other techniques of fecal examination in small animal practice are rarely required. Procedures which provide a measure of egg numbers are frequently unreliable and are usually not appropriate in small animal medicine. Sedimentation techniques for diagnosing fluke infections may be valuable if trematode species are suspected, but cannot be demonstrated by flotation or direct exams. Included here is a sedimentation test adapted from Dunn, 1978.

1. A three gram sample of feces is mixed thoroughly with water and the suspension is passed through a sieve with a mesh of 80/sq. inch.

2. The filtrate is collected into a conical glass container and sedimented for 5 minutes.

3. The supernatant is removed and further sedimentation is performed in a standard conical centrifuge tube. Washings of the sieve and glass container should also be added to the sample.

4. Following sedimentation, a drop of 1% methylene blue or parasitological iodine (see Appendix) can be added to the remaining fecal material.

5. Sedimented material is then poured into a petri dish and examined under a dissecting microscope. Examination of the material under a compound microscope requires tedious scanning of the sediment drop by drop and is not recommended.

In some cases adult worms are passed in the feces or vomitus or are discovered at necropsy and these may be preserved for later identification. Buffered formalin (see Appendix) is the best general fixative, but worms should be relaxed first in water for 10-15 minutes before being fixed. Parasites placed directly in formalin will contract and may become distorted and this makes it difficult to examine important features later. Use of alcohol as a fixative is not suggested, because it makes helminths brittle and they break easily on further handling.

For microscopic examination of important diagnostic features of adult worms, parasites may be placed on a slide in a drop of Hoyer's solution (see Appendix) overnight for clearance of soft tissue. The mouth and pharyngeal characteristics and the tail of nematodes usually provide the most useful diagnostic features. If necessary, heads and tails may be removed from the body of the worms for easier examination and clearance with Hoyer's solution. If mature flukes, tapeworms or female nematodes are available, the uterus can be ruptured to release ova or larvae. This often provides a rapid method of genus or species identification without resorting to other more elaborate morphological characteristics.

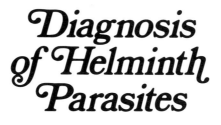

Diagnosis of Helminth Parasites

CESTODES

All of the cestode parasites which infect dogs and cats in the USA are transmitted *via* intermediate hosts. In the case of the taeniid tapeworms *(Taenia* spp, *Echinococcus* spp), the larval forms occur in the tissues of small mammals which are generally preyed upon by carnivores. *Dipylidium caninum*, on the other hand, is transmitted *via* the common dog and cat fleas *(Ctenocephalides* spp) or the biting louse *(Trichodectes)*. *Mesocestoides* has a more complicated cycle in which arthropods and then small vertebrates (birds, rodents) serve as intermediate hosts in transmission to dogs and cats. The much more unusual pseudophyllidean tapeworms *Diphyllobothrium* and *Spirometra* are generally restricted in their occurrence to the Great Lakes region of North America. Before establishing in the intestine of dogs or cats, and occasionally man, they pass firstly through free-living aquatic *Crustacea*, then into lower vertebrates (fish or frogs, respectively). These features of life cycles are important because knowledge of them can be helpful in diagnosis and management of cases of tapeworm infection.

PARASITOLOGIC DIAGNOSIS

Most often infection is diagnosed by the detection of proglottids, or segments, shed from the terminal part of the worm, and passed on or in the formed freshly passed stool (Figure 1). The creamy white fresh segments, washed or picked from the feces are quite active, especially those of *Dipylidium*. The characteristic shapes of each species may be difficult to discern until the specimens have been allowed to relax in water (Figure 2). Segments of *Dipylidium* may be up to 15mm in length and taper at both ends where they unite with one another to

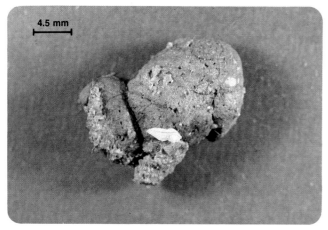

Fig. 1. Taeniid tapeworm segments on freshly passed stool. Proglottids are active when fresh but dry out quickly.

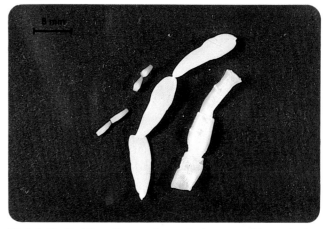

Fig. 2. Segments of the most commonly occurring tapeworms of dogs and cats. *Dipylidium* shows the characteristic taper at both ends, while those of *Taenia* have a more rectangular appearance. The small proglottids of *Mesocestoides* have a blunt triangular shape.

form the ribbon-like body of the tapeworm. *Taenia* spp proglottids are generally more rectangular in form than those of *Dipylidium*, and in ripe proglottids the creamy mass of eggs in the branched uterus can be seen grossly (Figure 3). However, the squirming movements of the segment both in the intestine and in the feces may result in the expression of all or most of the ova, and this appearance is therefore not always seen. In contrast to other members of the taeniid family of tapeworms, *Echinococcus* segments are very small (1-3 mm) and are unlikely to be detected unless they are sought by an experienced eye.

Mesocestoides proglottids are smaller than those of *Dipylidium* or *Taenia* spp, and are club-shaped (Figure 4). At one end a dense white spot marks the presence of a thick-walled uterine capsule. They are also quite active, and may quickly be dispersed from the surface of fecal deposits. The terminal segments of *Diphyllobothrium* and *Spirometra* are not shed routinely, but expel their eggs within the intestine while still attached to the worm. Periodically, long sections of the flat, rectangularly segmented worms are passed as they break off, but these may be completely devoid of eggs and are generally inactive or disintegrated.

Clients may frequently collect segments, either because they have seen them on the feces, or occasionally on the coat of the hindquarters of their dog or cat. Segments may even be deposited on furniture, carpets or clothing and cause alarm or concern, often being misidentified, when fresh, as maggots or as entire worms. Unless they are kept moist, proglottids quickly dry out and are presented as crumpled, white, leaf-like structures (Figure 5). They should be rehydrated, by soaking them in water for several hours, if they are to be identified accurately.

There is certainly justification for making the effort to arrive at an accurate diagnosis, despite the fact that most, though not all, of the commonly used cestocidal drugs are effective against a wide spectrum of different tapeworms. Further identification requires microscopy, under the low power, of segments placed in water and squashed between two slides or under a coverslip. There is no value in

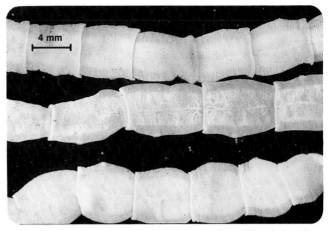

Fig. 3. Mature *Taenia* segments have a creamy mass of eggs filling the branches of the uterus. Each has a single reproductive system and one lateral pore. These pores may be very prominent in some species but on the most common taeniids in dogs *(T. pisiformis)* and cats *(T. taeniaeformis)*, they are not very noticeable. Often many eggs are expelled through the pore by the wriggling movements of the parasites as they move down the intestine and pass out with the feces.

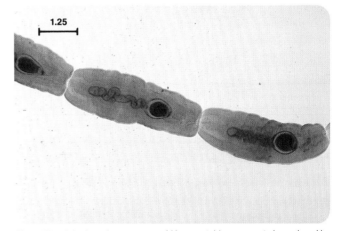

Fig. 4. The club-shaped appearance of *Mesocestoides* segments is produced by the tough uterine capsule at the terminal end of each proglottid. Unlike *Taenia* tapeworms, individual eggs are not released but remain inside the capsule.

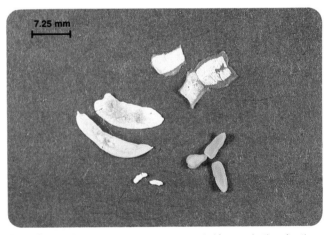

Fig. 5. Frequently tapeworm segments are presented for examination after they are dried. Although they may be difficult to identify in this condition, soaking them in water effectively restores their normal appearance.

examining dried specimens under the microscope. Water must be added or the diagnostic features are difficult to see. Segments of *Dipylidium* have a dual reproductive system and two pores (Figure 6), whereas those of *Taenia* spp have only a single reproductive system and, therefore, one pore (Figure 3). The pore itself may be more or less prominent depending on the species, though this is not an altogether reliable criterion for speciation. The single thick-walled uterine capsule of *Mesocestoides* is very characteristic, even at low magnification.

If the proglottids are damaged, the pores may not be very easy to see, and further examination of the contents of the segments may be necessary. This can be done by disrupting or crushing the segment with a needle or scalpel and placing fragments, or,

if the size permits, the entire proglottid, under a coverslip in water and examining it under higher power. At this point, the identification of the specimen as a cestode can be confirmed by the presence of the numerous calcareous mineral granules (Figure 7), which serve to distinguish tapeworm tissues from those of such things as arthropod larvae or earthworm fragments which may be present in the sample.

Eggs of *Dipylidium* are clustered in packets containing up to 20 eggs. These packets are readily recognizable both in the intact proglottid and after the segments have been crushed (Figure 8), whereas ova of *Taenia* spp are scattered in clumps or chains in the branches of the uterus. The eggs appear dense and brown in color (Figure 9). They contain a

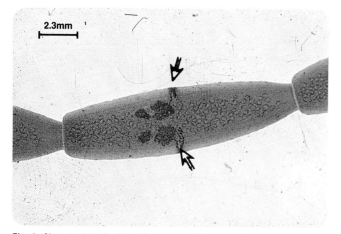

Fig. 6. Characteristically, *Dipylidium* segments have two independent reproductive systems and two pores (arrow). This is a very useful diagnostic feature in differentiating *Dipylidium* from other tapeworms.

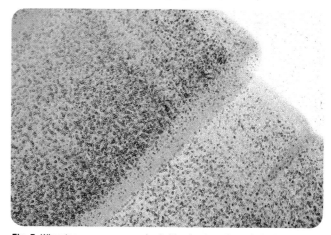

Fig. 7. When tapeworms are examined either fresh or after rehydration of dried segments, the numerous mineral granules are useful in differentiating them from other tissues and artefacts that may be present in dog and cat feces.

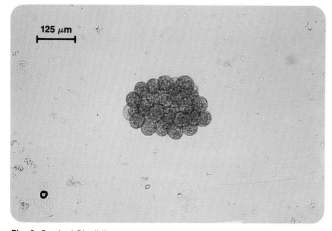

Fig. 8. Crushed *Dipylidium* segments release these egg-packets which fill the uterus of the mature proglottid. Egg packets may be up to 500 μm in length, and are diagnostic of *Dipylidium* infection.

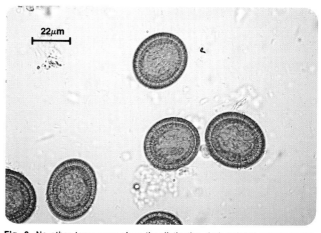

Fig. 9. No other tapeworms show the distinctive dark striated corona of the taeniid eggs. The corona is due to the tough radially-arranged blocks surrounding the six-hooked embryo within. Focusing up and down will show the radial arrangement best.

six-hooked (hexacanth) embryo within a striated shell or embryophore, surrounded by a delicate yolk cell (Figure 10). This six-hooked appearance is characteristic of all cestodes, and the embryo is commonly referred to as an oncosphere. If *Mesocestoides* segments are similarly crushed, the uterine capsule may rupture and the simple, shell-less embryos are released into the fluid (Figure 11).

The form of the egg packets or capsules of *Dipylidium* and the dense brown individual eggs of *Taenia* are also important characteristics if the diagnosis is made by examining feces using the flotation procedure (see page 4). Although individual proglottids, chains of segments or sometimes whole strobilae are passed in the feces and are the most reliable material for diagnosis, when these are unavailable, fecal material itself may contain individual *Dipylidium* (Figure 12) or taeniid eggs or egg packets of *Dipylidium* liberated from proglottids within the intestine. They float readily in most concentration solutions. In these preparations, taeniid eggs are no longer surrounded by the yolk cell which is usually digested away, but adherent fragments of it may roughen the outer surface. Taeniid eggs are small (about 30μ) and if they are to be identified and distinguished from artifacts, high power (40x objective) must be used.

By focusing up and down through the structure, one can detect the striation of the embryophore coat of *Taenia* eggs and the hooks of the embryo within (Figure 9). The eggs of all *Taenia* spp are very similar, and although those of *T. pisiformis*, for example, tend to be larger and more oval than those of *T. taeniaeformis*, the degree of variation makes it impossible to place much reliance on egg form as a means of speciation. The important point is that the thick outer layer with its characteristic sunburst appearance serves to distinguish them all from *Dipylidium*.

The diagnosis of infection with *Echinococcus granulosus* in the dog or *Echinococcus multilocularis* in the cat requires special mention. The occurrence of these tapeworms in the USA is not common, but their potential as human pathogens is cause for concern both to animal owners and veterinary personnel. If there is any suspicion that feces may contain

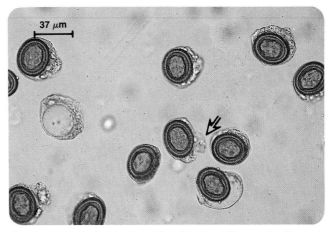

Fig. 10. Taeniid eggs freshly released from the segment have a yolk cell around them (arrow) but this is generally digested away during passage down the intestine.

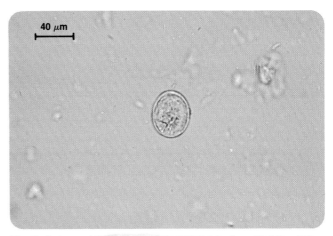

Fig. 11. Embryos of *Mesocestoides* are protected by the wall of the uterine capsule and really have no protective shell. If the capsule is ruptured, the fragile-looking embryos are liberated.

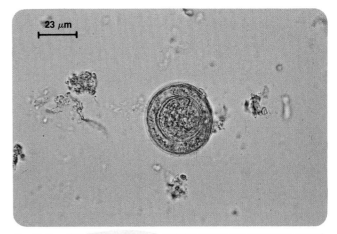

Fig. 12. Egg of *Dipylidium* has a thin shell with slight radial appearance around the hexacanth embryo.

eggs of *Echinococcus*, the sample should be boiled for 5 minutes before further examination. The segments, when passed naturally, are small (Figure 13) and fragile and unlikely to be detected. The eggs of *Echinococcus* are not reliably distinguishable from those of other taeniid tapeworms which have no significance as human pathogens. There are, in fact, no simple specific laboratory tests which can be applied to detect *Echinococcus* in animals in endemic areas of the USA, or even in animals which are imported into this country from highly endemic areas of the world. The only practical diagnostic procedure is to purge the animal with agents such as arecoline at 1-2 mg/kg which causes, within minutes, intense salivation (Figure 14) and vomiting, followed closely by extensive purgation (Figure 15) and passage of voluminous feces and mucus. All passed material including vomitus is examined by washing the sample through a series of mesh screens so as to trap the white worms or segments for final identification (Figure 16). The procedure is hazardous to dog and operator alike, but commonplace as a part of the diagnostic program for echinococcosis in many countries around the world.

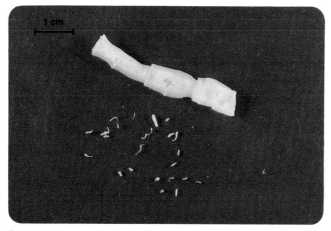

Fig. 13. These segments of *Echinococcus* are very small compared to those of the other tapeworms of dogs or cats. When infection is suspected extreme caution should be taken in handling and processing the sample.

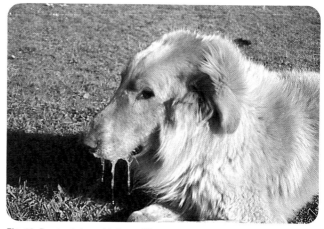

Fig. 14. Purging is brought about with arecoline at 2 mg/kg body wt. Most dogs will begin to salivate within a few minutes.

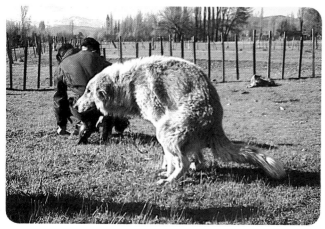

Fig. 15. Vomiting occurs shortly after arecoline administration, followed by passage of formed feces from the lower bowel, then *Echinococcus*-enriched small intestinal ingesta and mucus.

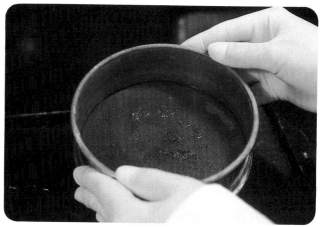

Fig. 16. All material being examined for *Echinococcus* must be regarded as hazardous. Protective clothing and gloves must be used and preferably fecal samples should be placed in boiling water for at least 5 minutes before examination. The sample is washed systematically through a sieve and the retained material examined against a black background for the tiny segments. All instruments should be sterilized by boiling or autoclaving after contamination. Even specimens preserved in formalin may contain viable eggs for several years.

The eggs of *Diphyllobothrium* and *Spirometra* are yellowish-brown and operculate, and must be differentiated from those of flukes by their size and shape (Figures 17-18). If parts of the strobilae are obtained, the squarish form and central pore are the most important diagnostic features (Figure 19).

Some pecularities of cestodes need to be emphasized from a diagnostic perspective. Firstly, the worms may survive in the gut for several years after reaching maturity, but do not shed segments constantly. The factors which affect shedding are not all known, but it is certainly unreasonable to expect them to appear daily. Infected animals may not pass any material of diagnostic value for days or even weeks. Secondly, eggs or egg capsules may be absent from the fecal mass even when freshly passed stools are covered with segments. In our experience, *Mesocestoides* embryos are never detectable in the feces, even in massive natural infections. Thirdly, the prepatent period is long, generally no less than 6 weeks for any species. It should be clear from these comments that the number of segments passed may be little indication of the number of tapeworms present or developing in the small intestine.

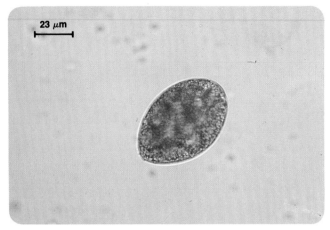

Fig. 17. *Diphyllobothrium* eggs are operculate and yellowish-brown with an overall length of 70 μm. The fully-formed hexacanth embryo will emerge about 10 days after passage by infected dogs.

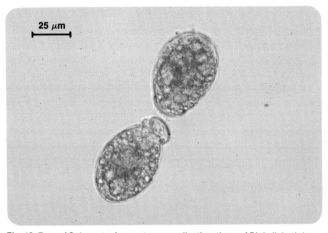

Fig. 18. Eggs of *Spirometra* from cats are smaller than those of *Diphyllobothrium* and more pointed. The overall length is 60 μm.

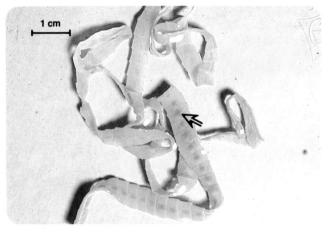

Fig. 19. The squarish segments of *pseudophyllidean* tapeworms (*Diphyllobothrium* or *Spirometra*) are often passed in ribbons, rather than singly, and each has a central pore (arrow) through which eggs are expelled.

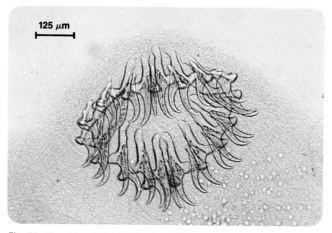

125 μm

Fig. 20. When the whole strobila of taeniid tapeworms is passed, the head should be examined for rings of hooks on the rostellum. The hooks are dagger-like in form with a handle, guard and blade. The length of the hooks ranges from 150 to 400 μm depending on species.

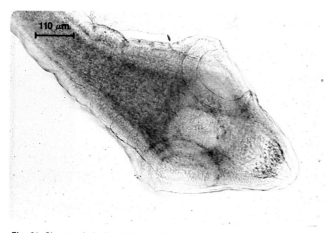

110 μm

Fig. 21. Characteristically, the head of *Dipylidium* has an armed rostellum but unlike *Taenia* spp. the thorn-shaped hooks are not arranged in rings.

It is also worth noting that other intercurrent intestinal disorders which produce hyperperistalsis, or even mild changes induced by abrupt alterations in diet, can result in the expulsion of long chains of segments or entire worms, including the scolex. In that event, examination of the head for the presence of the rostellum armed with rings of hooks for *Taenia* spp (Figure 20), the protrusible, finger-like rostellum with thorn-shaped hooks for *Dipylidium* (Figure 21), or the unarmed head of *Mesocestoides* (Figure 22) can be valuable. These features are also worth searching for in the fragments of worms, or whole worms, which are often passed after anthelmintic administration, if a complete diagnosis has not been arrived at prior to treatment. This may also be a useful practice to reveal mixed infections, which are not unusual, and may necessitate different kinds of advice on preventive practices for the owner. A final observation which derives from our own long-term study of experimentally infected cats is that during bouts of upper respiratory diseases, accompanied by pyrexia, dullness and anorexia, tapeworms may cease shedding proglottids only to begin again some days or weeks later when the animal recovers.

Those predator-prey relationships which lead to transmission of tapeworms also commonly lead to instances of pseudoparasitism which can be confusing. Rats, mice and rabbits are very frequently infected with their own adult intestinal tapeworms,

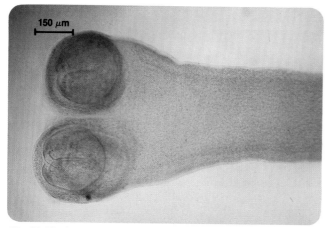

150 μm

Fig. 22. The head of *Mesocestoides* tapeworms is unarmed, in contrast to *Taenia* and *Dipylidium*. They do have the four muscular suckers typical of the more common *cyclophyllidean* tapeworms of dogs and cats.

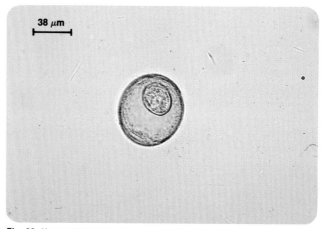

38 μm

Fig. 23. *Hymenolepis* eggs often appear in the feces of animals which eat rodents infected with adult tapeworms. The tapeworm embryo is surrounded by a large clear space and a smooth outer shell. The diameter is 55 μm.

especially *Hymenolepis* and *Cittotaenia* (Figures 23 and 24). Eggs of these worms pass undigested through the gut of cats and dogs and appear in their feces. Likewise, the coprophagic habits of dogs on farms often leads to the presence of *Moniezia* tapeworm eggs in their feces (Figure 25), especially in the summer months when segments of these prolific tapeworms are common in the feces of ruminants. *Hymenolepis*, by the way, may actively parasitize man, especially children, but this is in no way attributable to tapeworm infections in either cats or dogs. Despite this, they are often accused of being the source when a diagnosis of tapeworm infection is made in a child in a household with pets.

CLINICAL DIAGNOSIS AND SIGNIFICANCE

The importance of tapeworms as primary agents of disease in dogs and cats is difficult to assess, though this consideration has little impact on the demands made upon the veterinarian for diagnosis and effective treatment. By analogy with the experiences gained from human medicine, where gastrointestinal disturbances attributable to tapeworms are for the most part very mild, it seems unlikely that any of the commonly occurring tapeworms of dogs and cats in this country could be regarded as serious pathogens in infected animals. On the other hand, the bulky mass of worms in the gut may contribute to the intermittent disturbances in digestion

and motility, loss of condition and inappetence which are commonly attributed to tapeworm infections. The temptation to consider them as dietary competitors is great but over-emphasized, and only in the unusual instances of preferential uptake of vitamin B_{12} by *Diphyllobothrium* can one demonstrate evidence of specific nutrient deficiences in cestodiasis.

Nevertheless, from a practical perspective they are very significant because of their effects upon owners and, therefore, on the acceptability of companion animals as household pets. The passage of active squirming segments by cats and dogs is unsightly, distasteful, and repulsive to clients and their families, who understandably become concerned about their own health, as well as that of their pets. The irritation resulting from perianal movements of proglottids sometimes leads animals to rub or lick their hind quarters excessively and to a socially unacceptable degree, although this sign may be hard to differentiate from the problems caused by infection or impaction of the anal sacs. Objective evaluations of clinical consequences of cestodiasis are hard to come by, although it is clear from the experiences of investigators, including ourselves, who have maintained chronically infected animals, that in the absence of stress and given an adequate diet, heavily parasitized cats and dogs suffer no obvious deterioration in condition. However, accu-

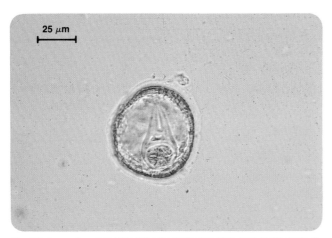

Fig. 24. Dogs allowed to hunt and eat rabbits may pass eggs of the common rabbit tapeworm *Cittotaenia*. These are typical of the anoplocephalid cestodes so common in herbivorous animals.

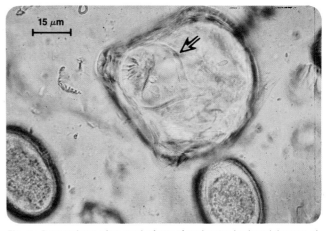

Fig. 25. Dogs on farms often eat the feces of ruminant animals and the eggs of *Moniezia*, the common tapeworm of cattle and sheep, may appear on fecal examination. The hexacanth embryo of these parasites is contained in a chitinous pyriform apparatus (arrow) surrounded by an irregularly-shaped outer shell. They are about 75 μm in diameter.

rate diagnosis is required of the responsible veterinary practitioner, and should be possible using the principles and features which we have illustrated, supplemented by other helpful information from the case history, and physical examination.

Infection with *Dipylidium* in the dog, and more rarely the cat, is indicative of the presence of flea or louse infestation. Treatment for elimination of the tapeworm must be done in conjunction with ectoparasite control, with appropriate attention, in the case of fleas, to the environmental phase of the life cycle. Dogs and cats become infected by ingesting fleas carrying the larval tapeworm, or cysticercoid. The larva is then liberated in the gut, and grows there to a strobilate adult form. Animals do not become immune and are readily reinfected if newly exposed to infected arthropods. Children occasionally acquire *D. caninum via* the same route, although the number of recorded cases is low, and almost all have been asymptomatic.

Taenia pisiformis is especially common in dogs which come from a rural setting where they may hunt rabbits carrying the larval forms, or cysticerci, in the liver and peritoneal cavity. Re-exposure leads to re-infection, and unless a complete diagnosis is made and the owner informed of the source, treatment may be considered unsatisfactory. Likewise, *T. hydatigena*, though far less common, occurs in rural dogs exposed to the viscera of home-slaughtered sheep, and occasionally cattle and hogs, which carry the cysticerci. A diagnosis of *T. ovis* implicates infected sheep meat as the source since the cysticerci only occur in striated muscle. This parasite is fortunately rare in the USA at this time.

Taenia taeniaeformis is by far the most common taeniid of cats (Figure 26). This is attributable to their rodent-hunting habits because the larval forms develop in the liver of mice and rats. A history of exposure to rodents, again especially common in a rural setting, is helpful in diagnosis and clearly important in determining the course of action for the owner.

The clinical significance of *Echinococcus* is entirely related to the infectivity of the eggs of these cestodes for humans. The larvae develop as cystic masses (hydatids) in the internal organs of susceptible intermediate hosts; normally sheep for *E. granulosus* in dogs, and rodents for *E. multilocularis* in cats. Hydatid cysts may develop in the liver, lungs, brain and other sites in humans, leading to chronic and debilitating diseases. Until recently echinococcosis, more commonly known as hydatidosis, was not considered seriously in veterinary practice in North America. However, the emergence of endemic foci of *E. granulosus* in several western states, and the spread of *E. multilocularis* from Canada down into most of the north central states, has led to some concern (Holmes *et al.*, 1970). Practitioners may encounter infected animals, especially in rural areas and, while they are unlikely to become involved in routine diagnosis, they should be alert to hazards of handling potentially infected animals or their feces.

Mesocestoides infections are often the result of bird or rodent-hunting habits of dogs, and though the life cycle is not completely understood, even dogs in an urban environment with sparrow-catching tendencies may be subject to infection. The tapeworms are peculiar in that they multiply within the gut and burdens of over a hundred adult worms may be found. Again, accuracy in diagnosis combined with a complete case history will lead to more effective advice to the client.

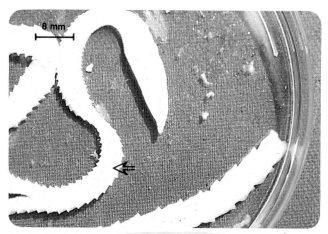

Fig. 26. *Taenia taeniaeformis* is the most common tapeworm of cats. Adult worms have a characteristic serrated edge (arrow) produced by the angular shape of the segments.

NEMATODES

Despite the development of a wide variety of anthelmintic agents which are effective against gastrointestinal nematodes in small animals, the frequency of infection with these parasites remains high, and a significant proportion of veterinary practice is concerned with diagnosis and treatment of roundworm, hookworm and whipworm infections. It is unlikely that prophylactic approaches based upon commercially available vaccines will be forthcoming in the near future. The construction of practical preventive strategies needs to be based on sound knowledge of the biology of these worms, on the limitations and advantages of anthelmintic agents, and on an appreciation of the finer points of diagnosis of infection and disease.

As with the cestodes, understanding the nature of the transmission pattern can be the key to successful laboratory and clinical diagnosis. This is especially true in the case of organisms such as the roundworms, *Toxocara canis* and *T. cati*, and the hookworms, *Ancylostoma caninum* and *A. tubaeforme*, because they have their most significant pathologic effects upon young susceptible animals in the neonatal period. These parasites have evolved efficient mechanisms to assure passage from one generation of hosts to another, and the resulting sequence of events offers a considerable challenge to the ingenuity of veterinarians and dog breeders alike.

PARASITOLOGIC DIAGNOSIS

Laboratory diagnosis of nematode infections is usually made by examination of feces for ova or larvae. Sometimes, especially with the stomachworms *Physaloptera*, and with the common roundworms, *Toxocara* sp and *Toxascaris leonina*, adult parasites are passed with vomitus which may be submitted to the laboratory for examination. This is particularly likely to occur after treatment with anthelmintics. Intestinal parasites may also be passed in vomitus following treatment for unrelated helminths. The heartworm preventative, diethylcarbamazine, for example, is an effective ascaricide and clients often see roundworms shortly after dogs begin DEC treatment. Alternatively, adult roundworms and whipworms *(Trichuris* sp) may be passed with the feces. In any of these cases, the gross morphologic features of the worms can be used for identification (Figures 27 and 28).

Progressing in order of frequency, the most commonly encountered nematode eggs in both dogs and cats are those of *Toxocara* sp and *Toxascaris leonina*. These are known collectively as ascarids, or "arrowhead" worms because of the winglike extension

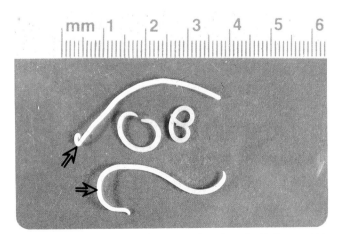

Fig. 27. Freshly-passed ascarids are seen here (arrow) with the common stomach worm *Physaloptera*. They have a creamy-yellow color and usually assume a C shape when they become inactive. Female worms are generally larger than males and may reach 18 cm in length in the case of *Toxocara*.

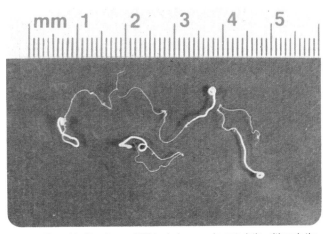

Fig. 28. The whip-like shape of *Trichuris* is very characteristic, although the common name of whipworm is a misnomer because the thicker end is the posterior part. Adults are usually several centimeters long, and female specimens may be up to 7 cm.

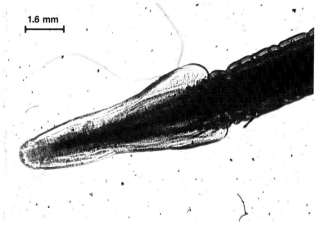

Fig. 29. Ascarid roundworms are often known as arrowhead worms because of the lateral wings of the cuticle alongside the head and neck region.

of the outer cuticle around the head and neck (Figure 29). Eggs of *Toxocara canis* (Figure 30) and *T. cati* (Figure 31) are passed in an unembryonated and non-infective form, and they require several weeks of development in the environment before larvation is completed (Figures 32-33). Consequently, only a single dense cell mass is seen within eggs in fresh samples, but the outer shell of all *Toxocara* eggs has a brownish-yellow proteinaceous coat which is finely stippled. Focusing up and down with the fine adjustment is the best way to detect this pattern, and the effort will be repaid by the ease of identification. The oval eggs of *Toxascaris leonina* are distinguished from those of *Toxocara* by their smooth surface and roughened internal layer, which is also

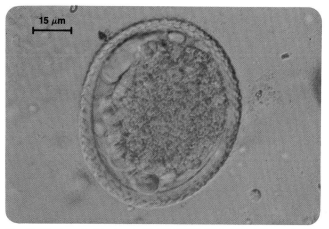

Fig. 30. The important feature in identification of *Toxocara canis* ova is the stippled exterior coat, which is best appreciated by varying the focus. The external diameter is approximately 80 μm. Fresh eggs contain a single cell as shown here.

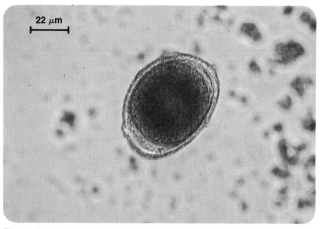

Fig. 31. *Toxocara cati* produces eggs which are slightly smaller (70 μm) than *T. canis* but the characteristically pitted outer coat is very similar.

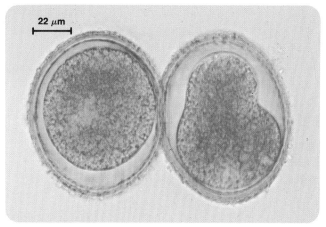

Fig. 32. Embryonation of *Toxocara* eggs involves firstly the division of the zygote into a dense cellular mass.

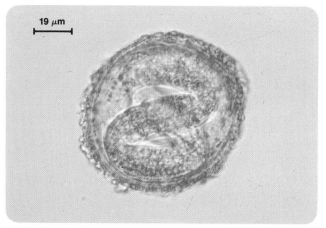

Fig. 33. The fully formed larvae of *Toxocara* will live within the egg for many months.

best detected by changing the focus (Figure 34). *Toxascaris* eggs embryonate rapidly and in a couple of days at room temperature the central mass of cells has formed a recognizable larva (Figure 35). Larvae often become very agitated during processing of the sample, and especially in the warmth of the microscope stage they may thrash wildly within the shell. Specimens sent in by mail will often have larvae within the eggs. It is worth remembering that the eggs of most roundworms, once embryonated, may contain viable, active larvae even after sitting for years in formalin preservatives.

Roundworms are prolific egg producers and eggs aberrant in shape or size and defective in outer coat characteristics are not unusual. Some of these eggs may cause confusion by their strange appearance (Figure 36). However, it is generally true that one egg is not apt to be the basis for a diagnosis. When in doubt one should continue examining the remainder of the slide in detail so as to find other eggs which are more normal in appearance.

Parasitologic diagnosis of ascarid infections, particularly in dogs, can be complicated when coprophagic dogs have access to farm animal feces. Horses and hogs are often parasitized by *Parascaris equorum* (Figure 37) or *Ascaris suum* (Figure 38), respectively, and their eggs may pass unaltered through the dog, appearing in large numbers on fecal flotation preparations.

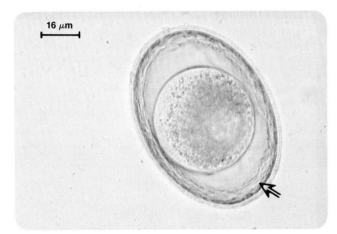

Fig. 34. The key feature of *Toxascaris leonina* eggs is the smooth outer shell and the roughened inner surface (arrow). They are generally slightly larger than *T. canis* and the overall length is 85-90 μm.

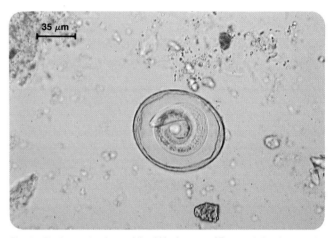

Fig. 35. The larvae develop rapidly within the eggs of *Toxascaris* but the smooth outer shell and inner roughened layer still serve to distinguish the eggs from those of other nematodes.

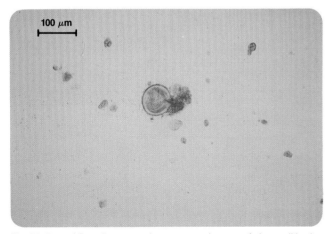

Fig. 36. Eggs of *T. canis* can vary in appearance because of abnormalities in shape or structure of the outer coat. Sometimes eggs rupture and spill their contents during processing of samples.

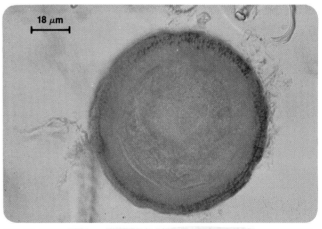

Fig. 37. Eggs of *Parascaris* may occur as pseudoparasites in dog feces. The heavy brown outer coat of eggs of *Parascaris* is an important feature in differentiating them from those of normal canine ascarids. They are about 90 μm in diameter.

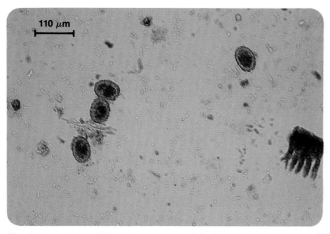

Fig. 38. *Ascaris suum* eggs have a characteristically corrugated rough outer coat. They are present in the feces of many hogs and coprophagy commonly occurs when dogs have access to hog manure. They are 70 μm in length.

The hookworms which infect dogs and cats are prolific and produce many thin-shelled unembryonated eggs typical of the strongyle group of nematodes (Figure 39). *Ancylostoma caninum* is certainly the most important in the dog because of its blood-sucking habits, but *Uncinaria stenocephala* (Figure 40) and *A. braziliense* can also cause enteric disease. In cats *A. tubaeforme* occurs most often (Figure 41) but cases of *U. stenocephala* have been reported. In fresh fecal samples, the detection of strongyle-type eggs presents little problem, but especially under warm and humid conditions, embryonation and hatching occur quickly. Active larvae then appear in flotation preparations (Figure 42), and this can cause confusion. Moreover, larvae

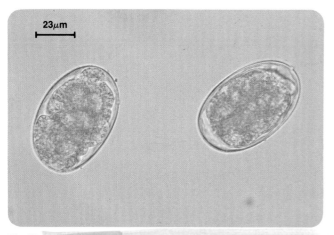

Fig. 39. Typical *Ancylostoma* hookworm eggs have a smooth, thin outer shell and contain several cells which quickly divide to form a morula, or cluster, after passage. Egg length is up to 75 μm and width 40-50 μm.

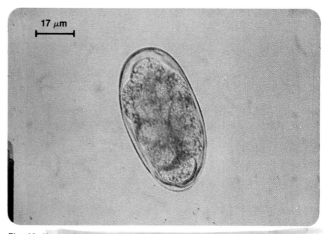

Fig. 40. *Uncinaria* eggs are very similar to *Ancylostoma*, and although slightly larger, they cannot readily be distinguished.

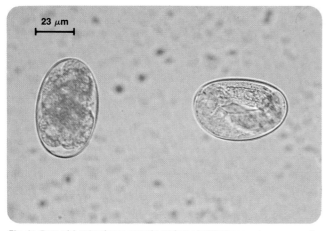

Fig. 41. Eggs of *A. tubaeforme* occur in cat feces but their general appearance is not distinct from that of *A. caninum* in dogs. The embryo forms within the egg equally quickly in this species.

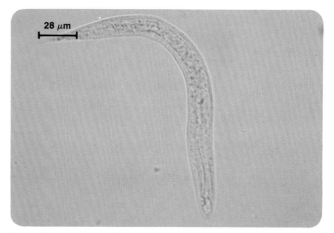

Fig. 42. Under optimal conditions first-stage larvae of hookworms hatch from the eggs in about 48 hours and may float up on fecal exams of old or stored samples. They are about 300 μm long.

sometimes die and become dehydrated and distorted to the point where they are hardly recognizable (Figure 43). The diagnostic problem is created by the fact that hatched hookworm larvae must be distinguished from those of *Strongyloides stercoralis*, (Figure 44), *Filaroides* sp (Figure 45) and *Angiostrongylus vasorum* (Figure 46) in the case of dogs, and *S. stercoralis* and *Aelurostrongylus* (Figure 47) in cats. *Filaroides*, *Angiostrongylus* and *Aelurostrongylus* occur in the respiratory system, but larvae are coughed up and swallowed and appear in the feces. The size of larvae and the anatomic features of the head and tail are key factors in differential diagnosis.

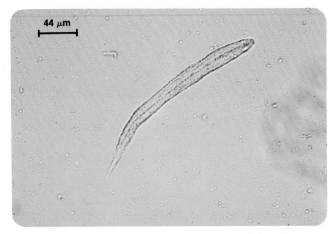

Fig. 43. Larvae may become desiccated by the flotation solution and are very distorted in appearance when they float up in fecal preparations.

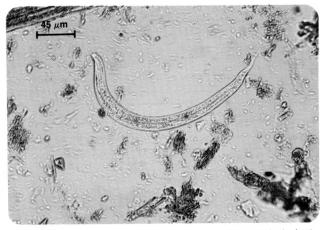

Fig. 44. *Strongyloides* larvae, rather than eggs, normally appear in the fresh feces of infected dogs.

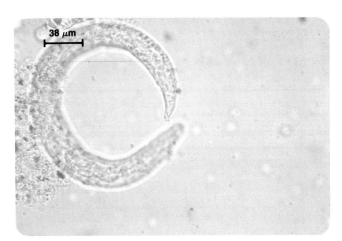

Fig. 45. Larvae of *Filaroides* are present in fresh feces of dogs infected with lung-worms but they have a very characteristic kinked tail which distinguishes them from hookworms or *Strongyloides*.

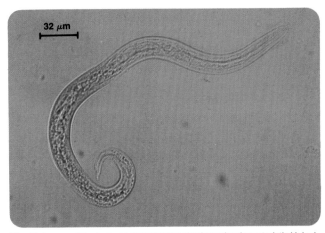

Fig. 46. Larvae of *Angiostrongylus vasorum* also have the characteristic kinked tail of metastrongyle (lungworm) larvae. These parasites are occasionally found in feces of dogs imported into the U.S.A. or in animals which have lived overseas in endemic areas.

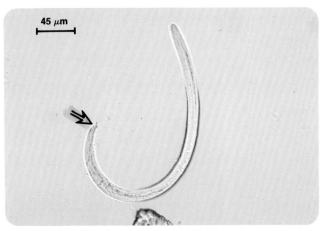

Fig. 47. Larvae in fresh feces of cats are most likely to be *Aelurostrongylus* (lungworms), because *Strongyloides* is extremely rare in the cat. These larvae show the kinked tail diagnostic of lungworms (arrow).

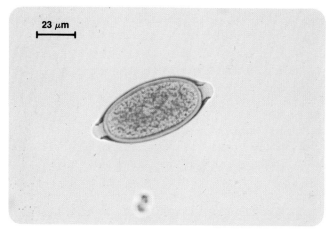

Fig. 48. *Trichuris vulpis*, the common whipworm of dogs, produces eggs which have a yellow or brown smooth outer coat, a symmetrical football shape and bipolar plugs. There is a granular mass inside but embryonated eggs are unlikely to be seen because larvae develop slowly over a period of several months in the environment. Their length is variable but generally is about 85 μm and width 40 μm.

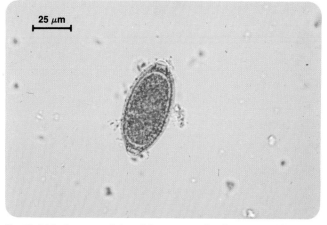

Fig. 49. *Trichuris campanula* is an infrequent parasite of cats in the U.S.A. The appearance of the egg is similar to that of *T. vulpis* in dogs.

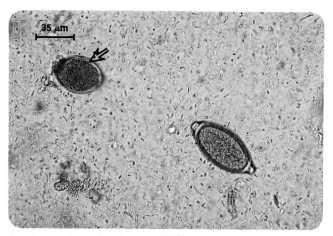

Fig. 50. The end-on- orientation of *Trichuris* eggs (arrow) disguises the characteristic bipolar plugs and may prevent identification.

Adult *Strongyloides stercoralis* are parasites of the small intestine where they release eggs that hatch immediately. Larvae are sometimes not demonstrable in feces, but may be detected in dogs in preparations obtained directly on a gloved finger rubbed along the rectal wall. Whether they reside there for any length of time or accumulate there for periodic bouts of shedding is not known. Larvae move actively in fresh feces mixed with saline and may be detected when present in large numbers by low power microscopic scanning of a fecal saline mixture. Alternatively, if their presence is suspected, a small lagoon of water surrounded by a rim of feces can be left at room temperature for a few hours. Larvae may swim into the central fluid region which is then sampled and scanned. Once again, flotation in hypertonic salt solutions may cause serious distortion.

Trichuris vulpis is the common whipworm of dogs, and *T. campanula* is the much more rare counterpart in cats. *Trichuris* eggs are unembryonated when passed and have a yellowish-brown color with a characteristic bipolar plug structure (Figures 48-49). Female worms are not as prolific as ascarids, but misshapen or fused pairs of eggs are often seen. The eggs float well in most concentrating solutions but occasionally become oriented end-on under the coverslip and their appearance can be deceptive. A slight nudge on the coverslip will usually cause them to flip upwards and lie with their long axis horizontally (Figure 50). In this position, the symmetry of the eggs is evident, and this is diagnostically important in distinguishing them from *Capillaria aerophila*. *Capillaria* live in the respiratory system and release eggs which are coughed up and swallowed and appear in the feces. The eggs are generally smaller than those of *Trichuris* and less pigmented, but most important, they have asymmetrically placed terminal plugs (Figure 51).

The only other plugged eggs liable to be present in dog feces are those derived from coprophagy of ruminant or hog feces containing *Trichuris* eggs specific to these hosts. The presence of other typical farm animal parasite eggs or oocysts in the sample will confirm that this has happened. Both cats and dogs which are keen hunters may show singly operculated eggs of rodent pinworms (Figure 52) which occasionally cause confusion. Less commonly one encounters *Capillaria hepatica* eggs which are released from adult *Capillaria* inhabiting the liver in wild rats.

It is worth emphasizing at this point that eggs of *Enterobius vermicularis* (Figure 53), the pinworm of humans, are occasionally found in the feces of dogs and cats in households where members of the family are infected. This is simply a reflection of the intensity of contamination of the environment within the household with pinworm eggs which then pass through the intestine of the pet after contamination

of the food or from licking the hands of infected children. Dogs and cats do not become infected with human pinworms despite the fact that they are frequently and unjustly accused of being at fault when pinworm problems surface in children.

The only nematodes parasitizing the gastrointestinal tract in small animals which produce fully embryonated eggs detectable in fresh feces are the spirurids. Parasites in this group typically inhabit the upper parts of the tract. *Physaloptera* spp occur in the stomach and duodenum, and *Spirocerca lupi* invades the esophagus and stomach wall. Each egg of these organisms is smooth-shelled, unpigmented

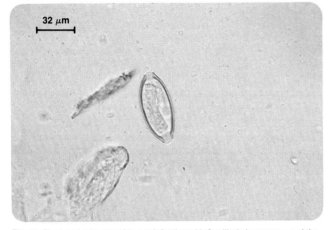

Fig. 51. Dogs and cats are subject to infection with *Capillaria* lungworms and the eggs which are passed are deceptively similar to those of *Trichuris*. However, *Capillaria* eggs have a stubbier barrel shape and paler color. If the eggs of *Capillaria* are oriented appropriately, the polar plugs can be shown to be asymmetrically placed. The overall length usually does not exceed 70 μm.

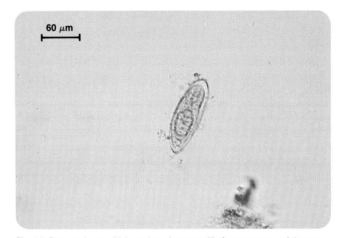

Fig. 52. Dogs and cats which are keen hunters will often pass eggs of the common pinworms present in the gut of mice and rats which they capture and eat. The eggs are usually asymmetrical in form and there is a single terminal plug or cap.

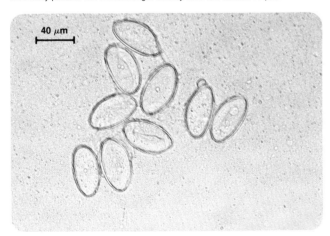

Fig. 53. Eggs of rodent pinworms are readily confused with those of *Enterobius*, the human pinworm, when seen in the feces of dogs and cats. Dogs and cats do not become infected with any species of pinworms and do not serve as a source of infection for humans.

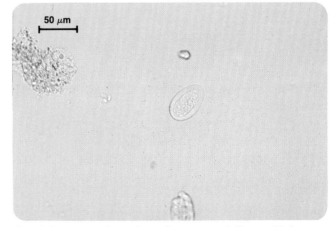

Fig. 54. *Physaloptera* (stomachworms) are very much like ascarids in gross appearance but their eggs are smooth-shelled and contain an embryo when passed in the feces. The diameter is about 55 μm.

and contains a larva (Figures 54-55). They are considerably more dense than most nematode eggs, and generally do not float well in commonly used concentration solutions such as NaCl or sucrose. Eggs of some species of *Physaloptera* do seem to float consistently in $ZnSO_4$ solutions (see Appendix), but dichromate solutions are necessary for serious attempts to survey for *Physaloptera* or *Spirocerca* infections.

Some general features of egg or larva production by gastro-intestinal nematodes are relevant to the effectiveness of parasitologic diagnostic procedures, and an awareness of these is essential for the clinical evaluation of enteric problems in dogs and cats. The prepatent period, for example, can be a time during which severe clinical problems develop, yet eggs or larvae are undetectable in the absence of mature female worms. Thus, puppies may acquire substantial burdens of *Toxocara* larvae while still in the uterus. Larvae sequestered in the tissues of the bitch pass to the pups in late pregnancy, though some evidently pass in the colostrum and milk. In kittens, passage through the mammary gland is the main way in which perinatal infections are acquired, but the clinical result is the same. Eggs may not be passed until the end of the third week of life, although immature worms may be voided with diarrheic feces or vomitus. Similarly, colostral transmission and, to a lesser extent, *in utero* transmission of hookworms, especially *Ancylostoma caninum*, can produce heavy infections in young animals which become patent during the second week of life.

An additional diagnostic complication arises from the fact that in adult dogs egg output may be intermittent or sporadic, and the occurrence of voluminous diarrhea may dilute the eggs and reduce the chances of detecting them. This necessitates repeated sampling to eliminate the possibility of pathogenic worm burdens, but it is hard to be definitive about the frequency with which this should be done. Some practitioners insist on three daily tests to confirm or deny the presence of hookworms, but cases occur in which clinical signs of hookworm

disease persist in animals which are fecal-negative for several weeks consecutively. The occurrence of this problem in northern zones in winter may indicate a seasonal influence on egg production by *Ancylostoma*, comparable to the situation reported in hookworm infection in man.

Trichuris has an extremely long prepatent period, up to three months, during which immature forms migrate into the wall of the bowel. The thickened terminal portion of adults then protrudes into the lumen. The pathogenic effects of the immature form have not been well studied, but adults can cause severe typhlitis and colitis. The opening of the cecum may even become closed by the thickening of the inflamed cecal wall. For unknown reasons, mature females may cease egg laying for weeks at a time and then, evidently in synchrony, return to production again. In these circumstances diagnosis by proctoscopy may be resorted to, and the terminal portions of the worms detected visibly.

In spirocercosis the problem is evidently not so much due to cyclic egg production by adult females as to the fact that the worms themselves become entrapped within the nodules in the esophagus and stomach, and eggs may not make their way into the lumen. Repeated examination may be necessary if they are to be detected in suspect cases.

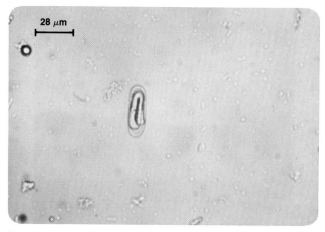

Fig. 55. *Spirocerca lupi* eggs contain a fully formed larva. They are by far the smallest of the embryonated ova seen in dog feces. The overall length is usually no greater than 40 μm. Eggs are often too dense to float in standard flotation solutions.

CLINICAL DIAGNOSIS AND SIGNIFICANCE

It is very difficult to point to a single well-characterized pathogenic mechanism whereby adult ascarids produce the clinical signs of mucoid diarrhea, poor growth, abdominal pain and abdominal enlargement (pot-bellied appearance), yet these signs frequently constitute the basis for the clinical diagnosis of ascariasis in young cats and dogs. The mass of the worms themselves may disrupt the passage of digesta leading to stasis, gas formation, changes in bacterial flora or hyperperistalsis (Figure 56). Chronic enteritis may lead to intussusception and thickening of the wall of the small intestine.

Direct transmission of *Toxocara via* the ingestion of infective eggs is particularly likely to occur in young susceptible animals and lead to the accumulation of large worm burdens. In heavily contaminated areas, the passage of large numbers of larvae from the gut to the liver and then lungs results in severe inflammatory changes in the respiratory system. These may in themselves be fatal or result in chronic stunting.

As dogs age, there is onset of a natural resistance which leads to many larvae failing to complete the lung migration and moving instead to the viscera and somatic muscles. These dormant or "hypobiotic" larvae in bitches form the reservoir for passage to fetuses and pups. Larvae acquired *in utero* may

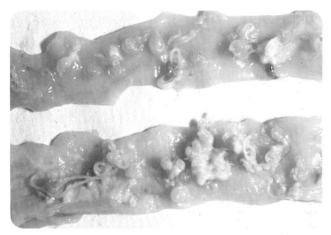

Fig. 56. Massive ascariasis often occurs in young dogs and cats and in some cases the bulk of the worms themselves leads to interference with passage of food, gas formation and chronic enteritis.

also cause serious problems as they migrate through the lungs, resulting in neonatal deaths.

Particularly puzzling to clients in these situations is the fact that mothers which produce such heavily parasitized litters appear themselves to be healthy and "parasite-free", with no detectable eggs on fecal examination. This anomaly results from the fact that adult animals exposed to infective eggs of *Toxocara* or larvae of *Ancylostoma* develop a burden of hypobiotic larvae in their tissues which are only stimulated to move to the uterus or mammary gland in the perinatal period. Parasitologic diagnosis in these females may prove negative because they do not necessarily have any mature parasites in their intestines. It is interesting that bitches may develop patent *T. canis* infections during lactation, though whether these derive from migration of some hypobiotic larvae to the gut, or if the bitches acquire larvae from the excreta or sputum of their own pups is not clear.

Adult dogs, however, can develop patent infections possibly from "trickle" exposure to the low number of eggs in the environment, or perhaps from hunting rodents in which larvae hatched from infective eggs have become sequestered. Under these circumstances, the larvae released from mouse tissues, for example, remain in the gut of the dog and mature without further migration. This mechanism is especially likely to occur in adult cats which are keen hunters.

Toxascaris occurs much less frequently than *Toxocara* spp, but can cause similar effects clinically. It also may be transmitted *via* rodents, although direct passage from dog to dog or even between cats and dogs does occur.

With the severest signs being encountered in young puppies and kittens, the clinical diagnostic problem of toxocariasis often focuses upon breeding establishments. Here an assessment of the management system, hygiene practices, treatment program for adult dogs, and rodent control efforts can all be helpful in confirming the diagnosis. An inspection of the premises at firsthand is the best way to achieve this.

Accompanying the problem of diagnosis of toxocariasis is the responsibility of the veterinarian in relation to human infection. Eggs of *Toxocara* are notoriously non-specific in their hatching requirements, and embryonated eggs will release larvae in the gut of most mammals including man. Thus, children exposed to large numbers of *Toxocara* eggs through ingestion of contaminated soil in the "dirt-eating" phase (usually 1-4 years) may develop a syndrome known as "visceral larva migrans" or VLM. This condition, and the related problem of toxocaral retinitis, clearly represents a link between parasitism in companion household pets and human health (Schantz and Glickman, 1978). Increased television and newspaper coverage of VLM has stimulated greater public interest in the problem and veterinarians should be in a position to make recommendations about sensible handling and hygenic practices to assist owners. Unfortunately, there is little information currently available on the epidemiology of VLM, making it difficult to identify the factors that increase risks of developing the disease. Actual contact with an infected animal has not been shown to be necessary. Surveys of public parks in Europe and the USA show *Toxocara* eggs to be common in soil samples, although the contribution of these eggs to the prevalence of the disease is unknown. Certainly active efforts by owners to prevent indiscriminate defecation by their pets may help to eliminate this potential source of infection. In addition, dog feces should be removed from children's play areas before the ova have become em-

bryonated and dispersed. Regular examination of pets and treatment of infected animals are also recommended to limit the number of infective ova contaminating the environment. Although most attention is focused on the public health importance of *Toxocara canis*, there is no reason why *T. cati* should not be involved and similar preventive practices employed. *Toxascaris*, on the other hand, does not migrate extensively and does not appear to be hazardous to man.

A very clear distinction needs to be drawn between the clinical diagnosis of hookworm disease and the parasitologic diagnosis of hookworm infection. For reasons which we have outlined, such as the intermittent output of eggs, the rapid development of eggs to larvae in the environment and the absence of eggs in the feces of bitches whose tissues are loaded with sequestered larvae, the demonstration of evidence of hookworm infection can be troublesome. However, the cardinal signs of hookworm disease are likely to occur in the great majority of cases in early life, and the development of marked immunity to hookworms more often than not leads to a balance in healthy adult dogs between their intestinal worm burdens and their immune response. Young animals are extremely susceptible to the blood-sucking habits of *Ancylostoma*. Evidence of anemia (Figure 57), weakness, dark-reddish brown or black hemorrhagic diarrhea (Figure 58), dehydration, malabsorption and wasting, should trigger suspicion of hookworm disease, even in the first week or so of

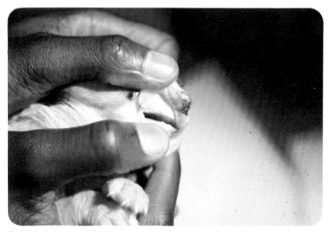

Fig. 57. Acute loss of blood caused by hookworms in suckling pups leads to pallor of all mucous membranes, weakness and death. Puppies may succumb to the infection before eggs are detectable in the feces.

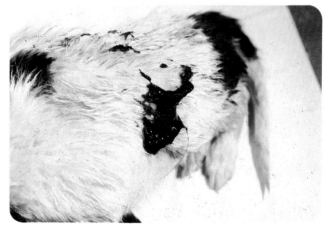

Fig. 58. Hookworm-infected pups pass chocolate-brown loose feces, characteristic of blood loss into the small intestine.

life when no eggs are being produced and shed by the parasites. Pups may eventually die of bloodloss anemia. Those hookworms which do not suck blood are capable of causing profound losses in fluid and plasma protein and this also can have marked effects on growth and performance of young pups. On the other hand, the onset of both a natural age resistance and an acquired immunity from initial experiences with *Ancylostoma*, make it less and less likely that subsequent exposures will lead to a similar sequence of clinical events. When they do occur, the key to management of the case is likely to lie in an accurate evaluation of the circumstances which determine the intensity of challenge.

Here again, the system under which the dog is maintained should be evaluated, so that the reasons behind the build-up of infective larvae to overwhelming levels can be understood. These may relate to overcrowding; poor hygienic practices which favor the accumulation of feces and, therefore, larvae; climatic factors which enhance the development and survival of larvae; soil or bedding characteristics which support the kind of microenvironment in which infective larvae can flourish; and intercurrent disease problems which may limit the effectiveness of the dog's defense responses. The collection of a complete case history is vital, and if breeding establishments, boarding kennels or laboratory animal colonies are involved, on-site inspection of facilities is essential for satisfactory management of hookworm disease. There is no doubt that the most profound problems are to be expected with *A. caninum*, but the pathogenic effects of *U. stenocephala* and *A. braziliense* in dogs, manifested as protein-losing enteropathy, can also be cause for concern when the challenge is allowed to exceed the capacity of the dog to react adequately.

An important factor in the immunobiology of hookworm infection is that larvae once sequestered are evidently able to avoid destruction by host defenses, and there appears to be no effective barrier to their subsequent activation at the end of gestation and wholesale migration to the mammary gland for transmission to the offspring. The immune response may also, in itself, be a contributing factor in the development of lesions. For example, a highly sensitized dog which is allergic to the antigen of the migrating parasites, may sometimes be suddenly or persistently exposed to skin penetration by large numbers of infective larvae. Under these circumstances, acute allergic reactions in the feet can result in intense pruritus, and even self-inflicted trauma as dogs lick and gnaw at their inflamed skin. Larvae migrating through the lungs probably cause respiratory difficulties in part because of the allergic reactions which are provoked in lung tissue.

This tendency to produce allergic reactions at the site of skin penetration is an important element in the public health significance of hookworms. Penetration of the skin of humans will occur, and, although the worms do not generally succeed in migrating past the skin, sensitization to subsequent exposure may occur. People who are habitually exposed (*e.g.*, animal caretakers, laborers on building sites contaminated by dog feces) can develop intensely pruritic reactions along the track left by migrating larvae which have penetrated exposed skin. This condition is known as "creeping eruption" or "cutaneous larva migrans".

Many of these comments on hookworm disease apply equally well to the diagnosis of strongyloidosis, although this condition has been much less well studied in dogs. Severe diarrhea, sometimes hemorrhagic and dark colored, may result in anemia, and can be produced by large numbers of *Strongyloides*. There is no clear evidence as yet of vertical transmission of this parasite in cats or dogs, but in other domestic animals passage through the milk is an important cause of neonatal strongyloidosis. It seems likely that this also occurs with *S. stercoralis*. The adult worms in the gut are parthenogenetic females, but the larvae they produce are capable of maturing into adult free-living males and females in the environment. These can reproduce and generate enormous populations of infective larvae which, like hookworms, penetrate intact skin. The potential for rapid spread and the accumulation of high challenge levels is clearly evident, and premises, even veterinary hospitals, where these worms gain a foothold can be very difficult to manage. The larvae will penetrate human skin readily and produce a tingling, itching sensation, though whether they can actually cause "creeping eruption" is not yet known. In some cases they succeed in migrating on through the lungs to the small intestine where they can produce clinical problems comparable to those seen in dogs.

Clinical trichuriasis is much more likely to be a chronic lingering problem, often without overt signs of intestinal disease, but resulting only in poor condition or performance. It does not follow the typical pattern of toxocariasis and ancylostomiasis in which young growing animals are severely affected and older animals become immune. *Trichuris* infections develop at all ages, occasionally reaching large enough numbers even in old dogs that they are shed in the feces and cause a fresh, and therefore bright red, bloody mucous coat to be voided with diarrheic feces. The worms do suck blood, though not as avidly as hookworms, and long standing infections can lead to anemia. Chronic gut irritation sometimes leads to intussusception, but rectal prolapse, which is so commonly associated with trichuriasis in man, is not characteristic of infection in dogs and cats.

Whipworms are acquired by mouth through the ingestion of embryonated eggs. The eggs themselves are remarkably durable and resist prolonged freezing. Although they may take up to 8 weeks to reach the infective stage, they can remain viable in the environment for years. They are virtually impossible to attack chemically, and the key to control on any premises is effective disposal of feces so that populations of infective eggs are not allowed to build-up. Desiccation and sunlight are the two key factors which need to be brought into play in trying to achieve this, and good drainage and aeration of pens and exercise runs is crucial. These measures, in combination with a program of anthelmintic treatment, are generally helpful. However, *Trichuris* evidently can persist in the cecum of infected animals even in the face of these efforts and surface as a problem once again in due course. It is one of the most difficult helminthiases to overcome satisfactorily. Incidentally, it has become clear that *T. campanula* does occur in cats in the USA and can cause similar clinical problems to those of *T. vulpis* in dogs.

The nematodes of the upper intestinal tract pose two very different problems. *Physaloptera* probably occurs with more frequency than is presently recorded, in part, because the eggs of most species do not float well, and in part because worms vomited up from the stomach or duodenum are very likely to be mistaken for ascarids. There is no question that their attachment to the wall of the stomach or intestine can result in irritation and excessive mucous secretion, and the sites of attachment become inflamed and chronically thickened. It seems likely that some cases of chronic digestive disturbances with intermittent vomiting, sometimes of bloody mucus, could be attributed to *Physaloptera* if the effort were made more often to reach a specific diagnosis. The requirement for arthropod vectors such as beetles and cockroaches, provides the key for adequate control of *Physaloptera* in kennels.

Spirocercosis can also result from the ingestion of infected arthropods, although more often insectivorous transport hosts (birds, rodents) come into the picture. The larvae hatch from ingested eggs and become sequestered and dormant in the tissues until this host is eaten by a dog. Then the larvae become activated to begin their complicated and long migration up the gastric blood vessels to the thoracic aorta, and then across to the wall of the esophagus or, less commonly, the stomach. The chronic inflammatory reaction which occurs there results in formation of a nodular mass which may interfere with passage of food into the stomach.

Clinically diagnostic features are the gradual onset of a regurgitative syndrome, with consequent loss of condition and malnutrition. The rate at which this progresses depends on the size of the nodule and its location, but the whole process may take months to years. The nodular mass may ulcerate so that anemia may develop as blood is persistently lost in regurgitated food or passed in the feces. Furthermore, there is a significant occurence of malignant transformation within the nodule leading to osteosarcoma or fibrosarcoma formation. These chronic pathologic changes lead to radiographically detectable dilation of the esophagus anterior to the obstruction, which itself may be visible in the case of advanced osteosarcomata.

Yet other complications of spirocercosis can occur which are important diagnostically. Damage to the aorta may result in chronic blood leakage or more often acute rupture and collapse, with respiratory difficulty, pallor and shock. The chronic changes resulting from the growth of space-occupying lesions in the thorax may lead to the condition of hypertrophic pulmonary osteopathy (Figure 59), though the pathogenic mechanism is not known. In addition, vertebral spondylitis may be associated with formation of the large mass. The entire complex of clinical signs may mimic those produced by foreign body obstructions, genetically determined esophageal dysfunctions or thoracic malignancies, and differential diagnosis can be difficult. The tiny eggs of *Spirocerca lupi* are not always detectable, and a knowledge of the incidence of the disease in the area can be helpful. The southern states of the USA are especially severely affected, but in the case of dogs which have travelled overseas and show this clinical picture, the development of spirocercosis should always be suspected.

Having diagnosed infection, treatment, especially in advanced cases, is very unsatisfactory. However, a knowledge of the origin of infection on a premises is helpful in designing preventive programs.

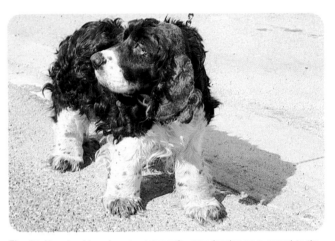

Fig. 59. Hypertrophic pulmonary osteopathy may develop as a sequel to the formation of large granulomatous masses around *Spirocerca* in the thoracic esophagus. Through an unknown mechanism new bone growth is deposited, particularly along bones of the forelimb.

TREMATODES

Intestinal flukes are not commonly associated with clinical disorders in dogs and cats in the USA but they do occur, and some features of their structure and transmission are relevant to the veterinary practitioner. Their life cycles are generally complex, involving passage first through a molluscan intermediate host followed by encystment in the tissues of some lower vertebrate which then falls prey to hunting dogs and cats. Once again, knowledge of the source of infection not only contributes to the diagnosis, but also affects the subsequent management of the case by the veterinarian and client.

PARASITOLOGIC DIAGNOSIS

All flukes are oviparous and their operculate eggs appear in the feces of infected animals. The organism most commonly encountered in North American dogs is *Alaria*, of which several distinct species are known. All produce large brownish-

yellow eggs which float in the commonly used concentration solutions employed for fecal examination (Figure 60). Fluke eggs, however, are quite delicate and often collapse and become distorted by the

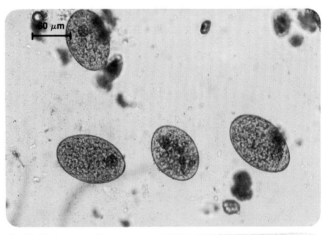

Fig. 60. *Alaria* sp. are the most common flukes of dogs in the U.S.A. The most characteristic features of the egg are its smooth yellow coat, large size (about 120 µm) and barely perceptible operculum.

hypertonicity of saturated salt solutions (Figure 61), and their appearance then may be troublesome diagnostically. They must be distinguished from the smaller, similarly colored eggs of *Paragonimus*, the lung fluke (Figure 62). Eggs of these parasites are released into the bronchial mucus and appear in the feces after being swallowed with the sputum. *Paragonimus* eggs also tend to collapse, but the shoulder-like ridge around the operculum is an important distinguishing characteristic.

Adult *Alaria* with their curiously divided body (Figure 63) are attached in the small intestine, and occasionally are passed entire, especially if the dog has diarrhea or is purged for other medical reasons.

If fecal samples are examined by sedimentation, rather than by flotation techniques, then care must be taken to distinguish *Alaria* eggs from those of other flukes which may have been present in the diet or prey of the dog. Ruminant liver fluke eggs for example (Figure 64) are not altered by passage through the intestine of dogs fed on liver containing *Fasciola hepatica*, and are strikingly similar to those of *Alaria*. The eggs of rabbit flukes also appear in the feces of hunting dogs, though they are small and readily distinguishable from *Alaria*.

Dogs in western states of the USA are subject to infection with *Nanophyetes salmincola*, larval forms of which occur in salmonid fish. The flukes them-

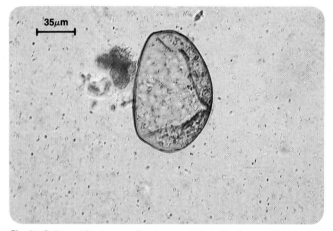

Fig. 61. Collapsed *Alaria* eggs often become distorted by the osmotic pressure of the solutions used for flotation. The shells buckle and fold and lose their smooth shape.

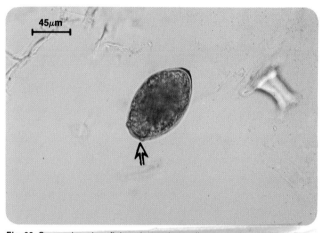

Fig. 62. *Paragonimus* lung flukes also produce yellow operculate eggs which are passed in the feces, but they are smaller than those of *Alaria* (about 90 μm) and the operculum is more apparent because of the ridges or "shoulders" (arrow) around its margin.

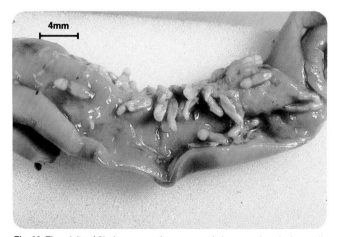

Fig. 63. The adults of *Alaria* are sometimes present in large numbers in the small intestine where they attach by means of sucker-like modification of the anterior end.

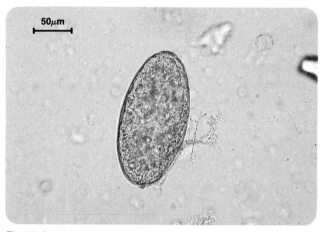

Fig. 64. Coprophagy by dogs in rural areas where liver flukes are endemic in ruminants can lead to the passage of the rough yellow operculate eggs of *Fasciola hepatica* in dog feces. They are difficult to distinguish from *Alaria* although they are slightly more tapered in shape.

selves are tiny (1.5 mm) and the eggs in the feces are brownish-yellow and operculate (Figure 65). Their significance as parasites lies in the fact that they carry a serious rickettsial pathogen, *Neorickettsia helminthoeca*, capable of causing fatal enteritis in dogs. This association with fish-eating has given rise to the term "salmon poisoning."

Cats are subject to infection with *Amphimerus felineus* which inhabits the bile ducts, and eggs are passed in the feces. It is of sporadic occurrence in central and northern US states, but more frequent in the southern regions.

CLINICAL DIAGNOSIS AND SIGNIFICANCE

It seems likely that most cases of *Alaria* infection are asymptomatic and go undiagnosed. There have been reports of mucoid enteritis associated with heavy infections, but their presence is most important as a complicating factor in the differential diagnosis of lung-fluke disease because of the similarity of their eggs to those of *Paragonimus*. Dogs probably acquire their infections by eating paratenic, or transport hosts, in which the parasite does not develop, but merely becomes sequestered and encysted as a mesocercaria. Rodents which eat frogs, the second natural intermediate host, may serve in this capacity. Some recent interesting reports implicate *Alaria* as a cause of serious systemic disease in man, presumably also by way of frog-eating

(Freeman *et al.*, 1976). The association between infection and rural hunting habits of dogs is an important one in advising the owner about reinfection if cases are diagnosed, though the history is liable to be similar in instances of paragonimiasis.

Amphimerus invades the bile ducts and occasionally pancreatic ducts in cats and may cause severe chronic inflammatory changes in each organ. However, the life cycle of this fluke is not presently known and it is difficult to construct an appropriate preventive strategy. It seems very likely that lower vertebrates or fish may be involved, though the possibility that rodents serve as transport hosts needs to be borne in mind.

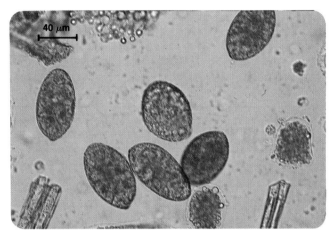

Fig. 65. Salmon-poisoning occurs in western states when dogs become infected with *Nanophyetes salmincola* flukes which carry a rickettsial pathogen. The eggs of this intestinal fluke are operculate and about 80 μm in length.

Diagnosis of Protozoan Parasites

FLAGELLATES

Flagellated protozoan parasites of dogs and cats differ from helminths in that they multiply within the gastrointestinal tract. Sometimes multiplication maintains low numbers of organisms which are barely detectable and probably non-pathogenic. On other occasions flagellates may proliferate beyond control, possibly in response to changes in diet, bacterial flora or host stress, and produce acute enteric diseases. This seems to be the pattern with *Giardia* and *Trichomonas*, both of which probably result in latent carrier states in infected cats and dogs, but occasionally appear as primary pathogens.

PARASITOLOGIC DIAGNOSIS

The vegetative multiplying forms, or trophozoites, of *Giardia canis* and *Giardia cati* occur in the lumen of the small intestine and attach to the surface of mucosal epithelial cells. In passage through the lower bowel they encyst and in clinical cases both the active trophozoites and the cystic forms may be detected in feces. Fresh fecal samples should be examined directly under high power by mixing with a small amount of saline on a slide. The whiplike action of the flagella gives them a jerky motion, though their mobility wanes rapidly after a few hours, especially if refrigerated. The characteristic face-like appearance produced by the ventral attachment area and the nuclei and nucleoli (Figure 66) can still be detected even in moving organisms, and if flotation concentration is done soon after collection of the specimen, recognizable trophozoites may be seen. More than likely, however, the more resistant cysts will surface (Figure 67), although the

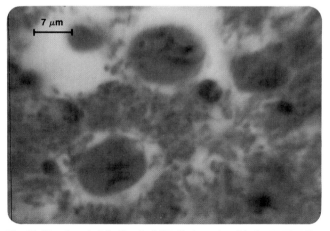

Fig. 66. The characteristic "face" of *Giardia* is produced in the cyst by the nucleus, nucleoli and centriole rod. These cysts have been stained in a fecal smear.

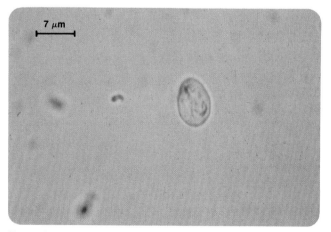

Fig. 67. Fresh cysts of *Giardia* show the thin, smooth outer cyst wall, and by focusing up and down one can see the internal structures. The length of these organisms is only about 12 μm.

hypertonicity of saturated salt or sugar solutions may distort these so that they assume a crescent-shape (Figure 68). Direct smears may also be dried and stained with Giemsa or Wright's stain (Figure 66) if there are doubts about the identity of motile protozoa seen in fresh saline diluted preparations.

Differentiation from the wobbling trophozoites of *Trichomonas (canis?)* is sometimes necessary in dogs. These protozoa have both flagellae and an undulating membrane (Figure 69) which ripples visibly as they move with a twirling motion. They are active only for a few hours after passage, and since no cystic stages are formed, examination of fresh feces is essential. In aged samples they deteriorate and become unrecognizable, but stained smears of fresh samples can be useful in identification. Occasionally non-parasitic protozoan flagellates of the intestinal tract are passed in the feces. Although these organisms give an impression of the rippling movement of *Trichomonas*, they are much smaller and cannot be easily examined for the characteristic undulating membrane of the parasite.

CLINICAL DIAGNOSIS AND SIGNIFICANCE

Low numbers of *Giardia* may be found in the feces of clinically normal puppies and kittens, but there is no doubt that they can also be overwhelming in certain cases and associated with severe watery diarrhea. Feces are often blood-tinged, and patients may become severely dehydrated. In older dogs a syndrome of less severe but persistent diarrhea is the rule, usually not sufficient to result in hemorrhage or dehydration, but in the longer run leading to poor digestion and loss of condition. *Giardia* spp occur in man and many other animals, and, although there is some evidence of interspecies transmission, the real zoonotic implications of infections in household pets are not known at this time.

Trichomonas in dogs causes characteristically an acute voluminous diarrhea with profound fluid loss, which may even be fatal if not treated both specifically with antiprotozoal agents and symptomatically for diarrhea and dehydration.

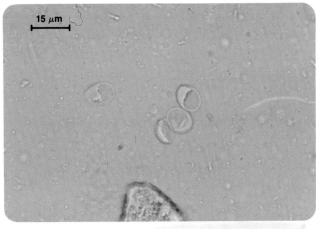

Fig. 68. *Giardia* cysts are frequently distorted by hypertonic flotation solutions. However, the distinctive refractile crescent shape of the collapsed cyst can be used to identify infection.

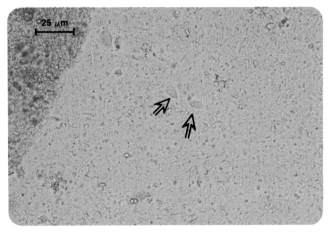

Fig. 69. The wobbling movements of *Trichomonas* trophozoites are best seen in fresh saline preparations. Rippling of the undulating membrane and flagellar movements are detectable by careful microscopy. The organisms are extremely small and delicate and cannot be preserved well (arrow).

CILIATES

Only one ciliated protozoan, *Balantidium coli*, occurs in the feces of dogs, and most infections are asymptomatic.

PARASITOLOGIC DIAGNOSIS

Trophozoites are large and very active in fresh samples, moving progressively with a smooth revolving motion due to the coordinated action of the many surface cilia. They have one very prominent nucleus, and a smaller, less conspicuous one, and may remain active for a number of hours, even when refrigerated, but they do not survive well overnight. Cysts form in the large bowel and will float in concentration solutions (Figure 70).

CLINICAL DIAGNOSIS AND SIGNIFICANCE

Balantidium evidently tends to associate with *Trichuris vulpis* in dogs, though whether the protozoa contribute to the pathogenesis of ill-thrift and diarrhea in dually-infected animals is not clear. It may be that changes occur in the bacterial flora in whipworm infections which favor the proliferation of *Balantidium*. In other host species, *B. coli* may become invasive and penetrate the colonic mucosa but this has not been described in dogs.

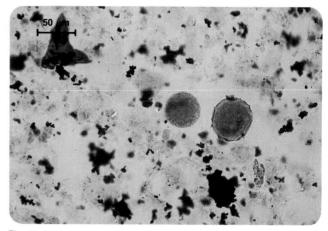

Fig. 70. The large (60 μm) cysts of *Balantidium coli* are usually seen in dog feces in conjunction with *Trichuris* infection.

AMEBAE

The simplest protozoan form is the ameba, and one pathogenic organism, *Entamoeba histolytica*, has been described in dogs. Dysentery caused by *E. histolytica* is a serious disease in man, and transmission between man and dogs is known to occur.

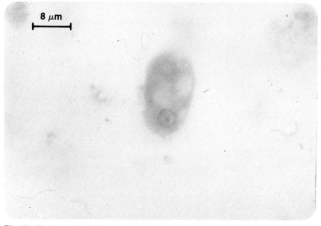

Fig. 71. Trophozoites of *Entamoeba* can be found in fresh dog feces and identified by the appearance of the nucleus which is characteristic for amebae. The organism sometimes becomes invasive causing severe dysentery.

PARASITOLOGIC DIAGNOSIS

Amebae proliferate by fission and trophozoites occur in the lumen of the large bowel. They do not usually encyst in dogs, as they do in man, so that microscopic examination of fresh or stained smears is necessary to reach a diagnosis, although by no means all cases are symptomatic. Active trophozoites moving by pseudopod formation can be seen in fresh saline preparations, and examination of stained smears reveals phagocytic vacuoles and the nucleus typical of this species (Figure 71).

CLINICAL DIAGNOSIS AND SIGNIFICANCE

Latent infections may be encountered as incidental findings in routine examination of fresh feces from dogs, but some animals develop severe hemorrhagic enteritis. Invasion of the gut mucosa and internal viscera, comparable to the syndrome in man, has been reported in dogs in the USA, but probably most cases of the intestinal form go undetected. Invasiveness may be related to changes in bacterial flora so that symptomatic treatment of enteritis with antibiotics may reverse the signs of *E. histolytica* infection. When cases are diagnosed, awareness of their potential for infecting humans requires treatment with antiprotozoals. Although described in other countries, amebiasis does not seem to occur in cats in North America.

COCCIDIA

The classification and identification of coccidia which infect the intestine of dogs and cats has become a fast-moving and controversial field. This has come about from the realization in recent years that many organisms not formerly considered to be related to the coccidia actually have coccidian-type life cycles. Furthermore, the life cycles of the classically known species of the dog and cat have undergone revision in the light of new research findings indicating that most *Isospora* can be transmitted *via* a two-host predator-prey pattern, as well as *via* the direct fecal-oral route. Compounding the diagnostic problem further is the fact that many of the species release small and morphologically identical cystic forms in the feces, which can only be differentiated by means of laboratory animal inoculation experiments.

PARASITOLOGIC DIAGNOSIS

In the main, protozoan parasites in this group proliferate in the cells of the intestinal epithelium or *lamina propria* and through a series of multiplicative phases, both asexual and sexual, zygotes are produced. These appear in cystic form in the feces. In some species, development is rapid once the organisms are shed, and the collection of fresh samples is a prerequisite. They float in most concentrating solutions and examination under high power reveals the refractile cyst wall surrounding the zygote cell (Figure 72). In the case of *Isospora felis*, the zygote rapidly divides into sporocysts containing sporozoites (Figure 73). Comparable species in the dog are *Isospora canis* and *I. rivolta*. The sizes of oocysts are most important in identification, although in most practical instances absolute identification of species will be impossible.

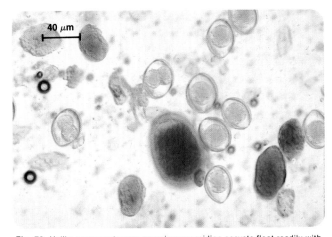

Fig. 72. Unlike many protozoan organisms coccidian oocysts float readily with little distortion in most flotation solutions. Unfortunately, the oocysts of many coccidia species are so similar in appearance that accurate identification is impossible.

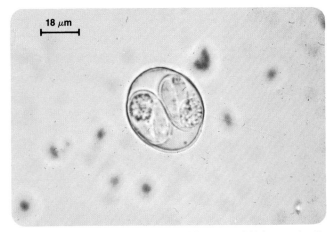

Fig. 73. The process of sporulation with coccidia occurs quickly in warm, humid conditions and the sporocysts can form in 24-28 hours in feces.

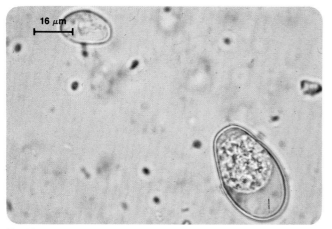

Fig. 74. Although oocysts of the *Eimeria* type occur in dogs, their pathogenicity is not known. The elongated shape, yellowish color and development into four sporocysts distinguish them from the more common *Isospora* species.

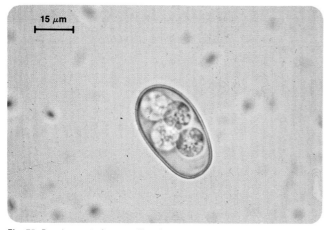

Fig. 75. Development of mature *Eimeria* sporocysts is preceded by division of the intact single cell of the oocyst into four cells.

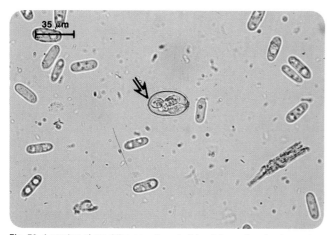

Fig. 76. A number of coccidian parasites of wild and domestic animals may be found in the feces of predators or coprophagous cats and dogs. The oocysts of rabbit coccidia occur as contamination of the feces of rural cats and dogs.

Oocysts of the *Eimeria* type (Figures 74-75) occur occasionally in the feces of dogs but their significance as causes of disease is not clear, and their identities are not well established. Diagnostic difficulties may also arise because of the passage of coccidian oocysts from other species, especially herbivores, all the way through the gastrointestinal tract. Thus, coccidia ingested with the tissues of hunted rabbits (Figure 76) or in the feces of cattle or sheep (Figure 77), which are often devoured by dogs, may appear on fecal examination of rural or hunting animals.

The tiny (10-12μ) oocysts of *Toxoplasma gondii* occur in the cat only, but are not distinguishable from other related species of *Isospora*, *Besnoitia*, or *Hammondia* (Figure 78), all of which may have similar life cycles involving predator-prey relationships. Serologic tests have been developed as an aid in the diagnosis of intestinal toxoplasmosis in cats, but the results have been difficult to interpret and the procedure is not widely used at present. Sporocysts (Figure 79) released into the feces of both dogs and cats infected with a variety of species of *Sarcocystis* are also indistinguishable morphologically, and must be fed to test animals experimentally for speciation. Sometimes sporocysts and small oocysts become slightly more easy to detect when flotation preparations are left for a few days before microscopic examination.

CLINICAL DIAGNOSIS AND SIGNIFICANCE

Coccidian oocysts are not shed constantly, and there is a great tendency for older asymptomatic cats and dogs to shed small numbers, perhaps periodically or under stress, so that they serve as chronic carriers. In fact, puppies and kittens may also acquire infection without the onset of clinical signs, and enteric disease may be difficult to reproduce experimentally. However, practitioners encounter clinical syndromes in young animals associated with extensive hemorrhagic diarrhea and constant straining, abdominal pain, dehydration, stunting and loss of body weight and hair condition, progressing to weakness and prostration. These cases may have abundant oocysts of *Isospora* in their feces on examination. Although recovery may occur, clinical experience suggests that not all recovered animals will remain as inapparent chronically infected carriers; some animals suffer repeated relapses with a similar set of clinical signs and respond once again to specific anticoccidial treatment and symptomatic support therapy.

The number of oocysts need not be high to establish a diagnosis of clinical coccidiosis in such instances, although where oocysts are present and clinical signs are absent, it is difficult to justify any kind of therapeutic intervention.

It is highly likely that the outcome of a puppy's or kitten's first encounter with coccidian pathogens is determined by the size of the initial infecting dose. Accordingly, in conditions where oocyst populations are allowed to build up, such as in the humid summer months in exercise pens, or even indoors in boarding kennels or breeding establishments, high infective doses may prove lethal. Under these circumstances, a visit to the premises where the problem has arisen can be invaluable, both in establishing the diagnosis, and in developing an effective preventive program for the owner or client.

It is unlikely that the veterinarian will encounter clinical problems associated with intestinal infection with *Toxoplasma gondii* in cats or *Sarcocystis* or *Hammondia* spp in cats and dogs. Experimentally these organisms produce, at worst, only mild clinical disorders. Their significance lies in the fact that oocysts and sporocysts may be infective for domestic food animals, and also for humans, in the case of *T. gondii* and some *Sarcocystis* spp. In fact, diagnosis of these infections is not likely to occur frequently on fecal examinations because the cystic forms are generally released only transiently. If they are released for longer periods, then numbers are likely to be low.

The responsibility of the veterinarian regarding *Toxoplasma* and *Sarcocystis* infections lies in the area of providing advice on the kinds of reasonable and appropriate preventive measures which clients should take. There are certain known hazards associated with toxoplasmosis. The most important of these is prenatal infection of children leading to congenital abnormalities of the nervous system. In addition, a flu-like syndrome may develop in indi-

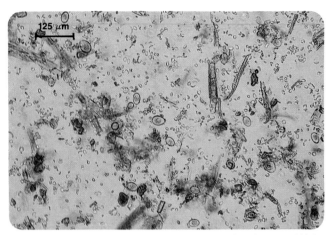

Fig. 77. *Eimeria* species are also common parasites of ruminants and birds. These ruminant coccidia oocysts from goats may be easily mistaken for those of cats and dogs.

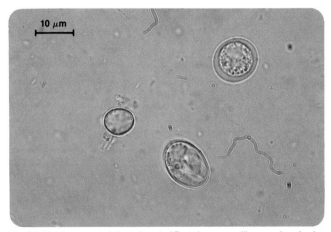

Fig. 78. The tiny oocysts (about 12 μm) of *Toxoplasma gondii* are produced only in cats. Although only a single cell is present in freshly passed oocysts, sporocysts can form in as little as 24 hours. Other related coccidia such as *Hammondia* species of cats and dogs produce oocysts which are indistinguishable from one another and from *T. gondii.*

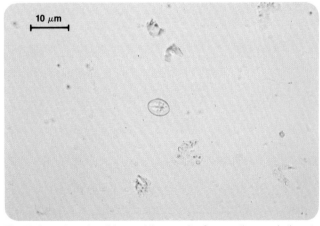

Fig. 79. Several species of the coccidian parasite, *Sarcocystis*, occur in the gut of dogs and cats. Oocysts are not passed but break down in the gut to release sporocysts, shown here. These tiny structures are difficult to detect in flotation preparations.

viduals first exposed as adults to *Toxoplasma*. However, serologic surveys indicate that many millions of people are infected without showing any clinical signs. When illness does develop in adults, it is quite likely to result from eating undercooked meat containing *Toxoplasma* cysts rather than from direct ingestion of oocysts passed by cats. On the other hand, in a household where there is a pregnant woman, some risk can be identified and it is reasonable to suggest that precautions be taken. The task of cleaning the litter box, in particular, should be given to another member of the family, and the litter should be changed every day before oocysts can sporulate and become infective. Hygiene is extremely important, and the person handling cat feces should wash his or her hands thoroughly. Cats which are kept indoors are much less likely to be a hazard. In addition to avoiding oocysts in cat feces, a pregnant woman should avoid eating rare meat and should wash her hands thoroughly after preparation of raw meat (Dubey, 1976).

The importance of *Sarcocystis* infections is not yet well defined. Human infection with the cysts of *Sarcocystis* spp is very rare, and there appears to be little chance of zoonotic transmission of those species commonly infecting dogs and cats. However, it is now evident that some of the species infecting pets pass through other domesticated animals in their intermediate stages of development. During the period of active multiplication in these hosts, *Sarcocystis* spp may cause fatal disease or abortion, and their importance as pathogens of domestic animals may require re-evaluation in the next few years.

Comparison of Parasites and Pseudoparasites

PSEUDOPARASITES

The following twelve figures are examples of the variety of artefacts which are easily confused with parasite eggs, oocysts and larvae in fecal preparations. A discussion of some of the general principles used in identifying these pseudoparasites is contained in Chapter 2.

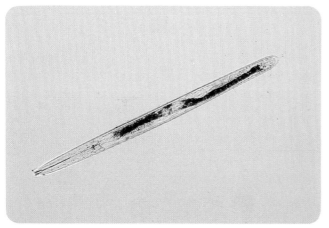

Fig. 80. Free-living nematode.

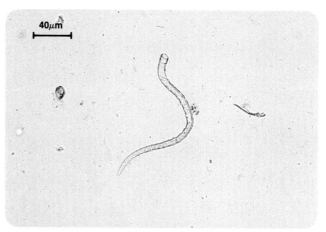

Fig. 81. Plant hair.

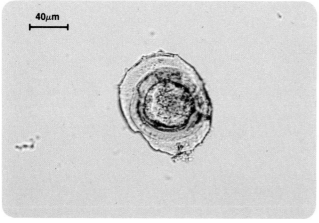

Fig. 82. Plant material.

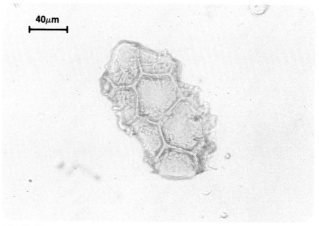

Fig. 83. Plant material.

CHAPTER 5

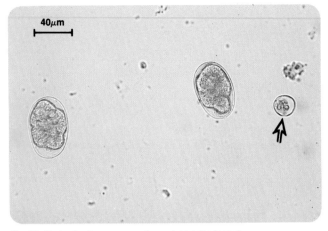

Fig. 84. Canine hookworm egg and pseudoparasite (arrow).

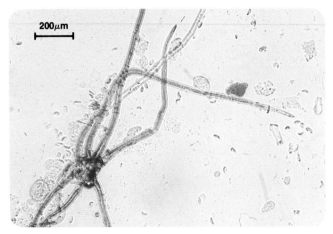

Fig. 85. Plant hair.

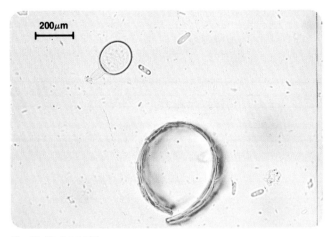

Fig. 86. Plant material.

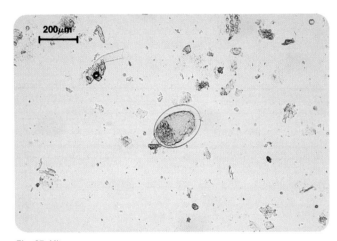

Fig. 87. Mite egg.

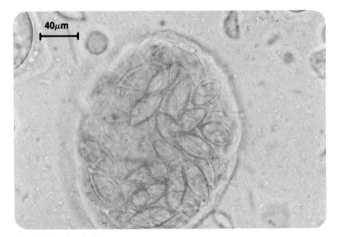

Fig. 88. Plant material.

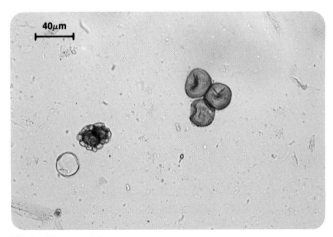

Fig. 89. Plant material.

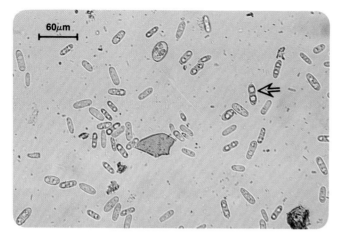

Fig. 90. Nonpathogenic yeast (arrow) and coccidian oocyst.

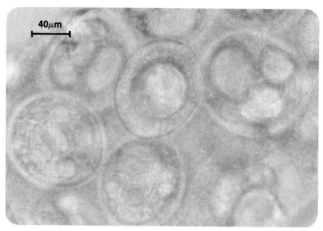

Fig. 91. Plant material.

COMPARISON OF PARASITES

An awareness of the relative sizes of parasitic ova and oocysts is extremely helpful in identifying these structures. Such comparisons are probably most easily appreciated when ova of several species can be seen in the same microscopic field.

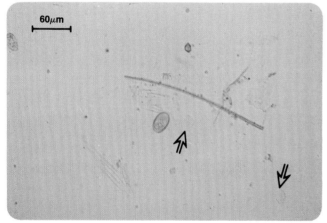

Fig. 92. Coccidian oocyst and Giardia cyst. (arrows)

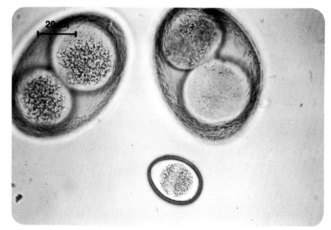

Fig. 93. Coccidian oocyst and *Toxascaris leonina* ovum.

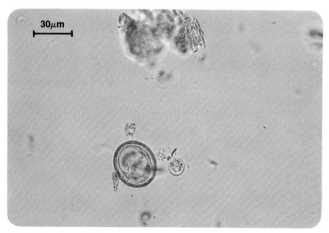

Fig. 94. Canine coccidian oocyst and *Taenia taeniaeformis* ovum.

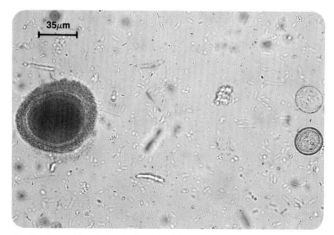

Fig. 95. Eggs of *Taenia taeniaeformis* and *Toxocara canis*.

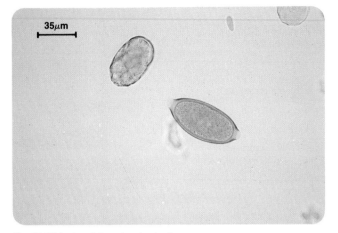

Fig. 96. *Trichuris vulpis* and canine hookworm eggs.

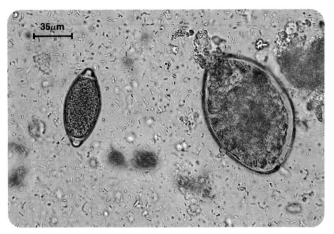

Fig. 97. Eggs of *Trichuris vulpis* and *Alaria* sp.

Appendix 1
Relative Sizes of Diagnostically Important Parasites

The composite illustrations on the following pages depict the most common parasite eggs on an accurate scale basis.

Relative Sizes of Diagnostically

All illustrations on pages 44, 45, and 46 are drawn to scale. |—| 20 μm

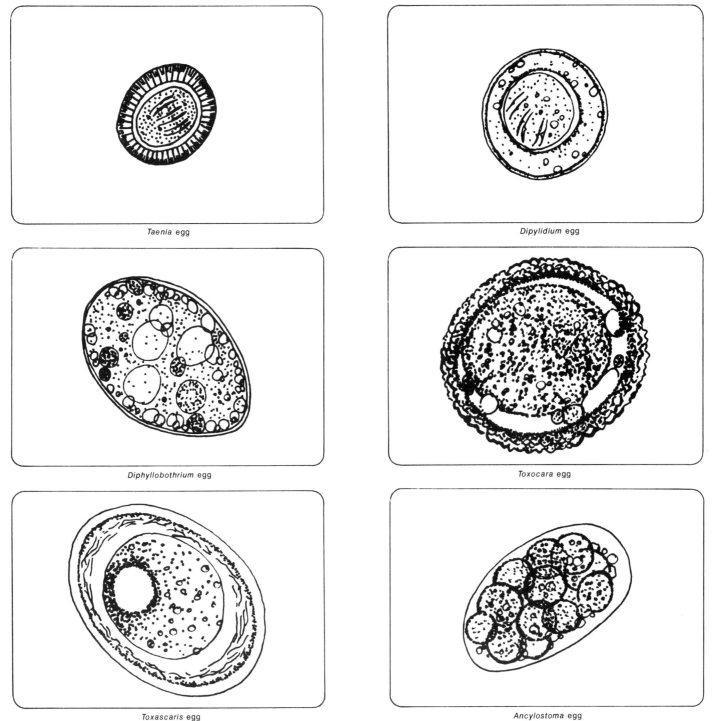

Taenia egg

Dipylidium egg

Diphyllobothrium egg

Toxocara egg

Toxascaris egg

Ancylostoma egg

Important Parasites

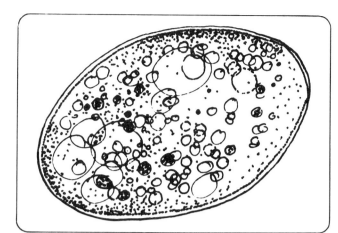

Alaria egg

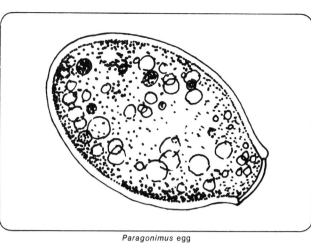

Paragonimus egg

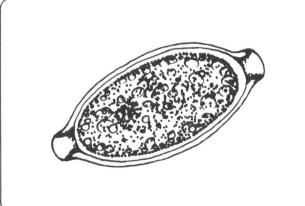

Strongyloides larva

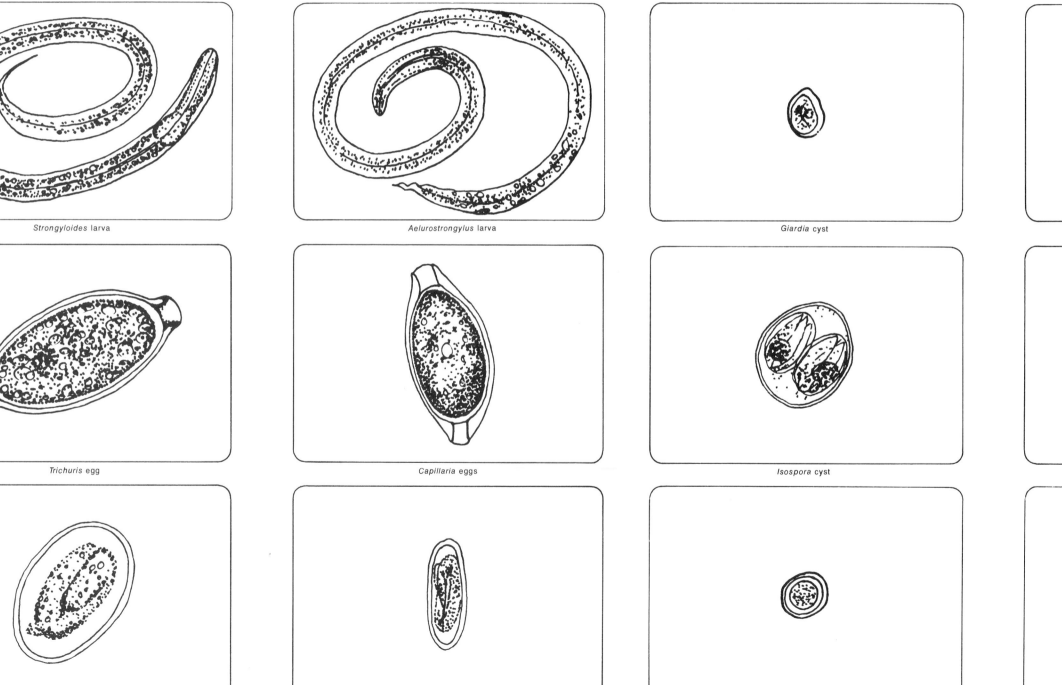

Aelurostrongylus larva

Giardia cyst

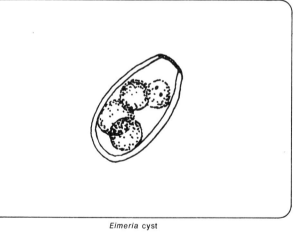

Balantidium cyst

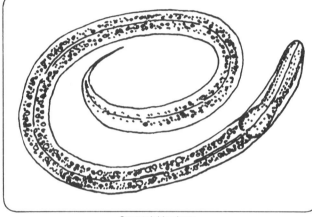

Trichuris egg

Capillaria eggs

Isospora cyst

Eimeria cyst

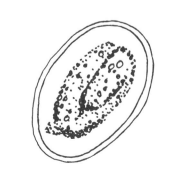

Physaloptera egg

Spirocerca egg

Toxoplasma cyst

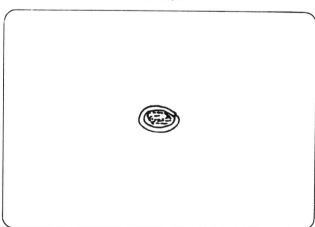

Sarcocystis cyst

45

Appendix 2

Reagents and Flotation Solutions Used in Diagnostic Procedures

REAGENTS

10% Buffered Formalin

37-40% formalin (commercially available solution)	100	ml
Distilled water	900	ml
NaH_2PO_4 (monobasic)	4	g
Na_2HPO_4 (dibasic)	6.5	g

For preservation of feces, the addition of the salts is not essential. However, buffered formalin is preferred for fixing helminth specimens.

Lugol's Iodine

Iodine crystals	5	g
Potassium iodide	10	g
Distilled water	100	ml

To prevent overstaining, the solution should be diluted several times before using.

Hoyer's Solution

Gum arabic	30	g
Glycerol	16	ml
Chloral hydrate	200	g
Distilled water	50	ml

Dissolve the gum arabic in water with gentle heat. Add the chloral hydrate, then glycerol.

Giemsa's Stain (Stock Solution)

Giemsa stain	0.75	g
Glycerol	25	ml
Absolute methanol	75	ml

The glycerol and stain are mixed until a paste is formed and then combined with the methanol. This stock solution should be stored in a dark bottle.

To stain fecal smears, the slide is dried and fixed in absolute methanol for several minutes. The Giemsa stain should be freshly prepared as a 1 in 10 dilution with buffered water (pH 7.2) and poured over the slide, which is allowed to stand for 30 minutes. The slide is then washed with buffered water, dried and examined.

Buffered water

Distilled water 1000   ml
Na_2HPO_4 . . . . 25.2   g
KH_2PO_4 . . . . 12.5   g

Wright's Stain

Undiluted commercial stain is placed on the slide for 5 to 20 minutes, rinsed off, and the slide dried and examined.

FLOTATION SOLUTIONS

Zinc Sulfate (33%)

Specific gravity 1.180

33 grams of anhydrous $ZnSO_4$ should be dissolved in and brought up to 100 ml with distilled water. Although a fully saturated $ZnSO_4$ solution is approximately 38%, the 33% solution is most frequently used because it produces less distortion of parasite ova and cysts.

Sucrose
(Sheather's Solution)

Specific gravity 1.117-1.3

Sucrose 500   g
Water 360   ml
Phenol . . . . 6.6   ml

The sucrose should be dissolved in water over indirect heat.

Magnesium Sulfate (35%)

Specific gravity 1.28

35 g of $MgSO_4$ is dissolved in and brought up to 100 ml with distilled water.

Sodium Chloride

The quantity of NaCl required to saturate water will vary with environmental conditions and consequently the specific gravity of a stock solution kept in the laboratory will also change. Generally, about 36 g of NaCl, which is dissolved in and brought up to 100 ml with water, will be needed to produce a saturated solution with a specific gravity of 1.2.

References

Adam, K. M. G., Paul, J., and Zaman, V. (1971). *Medical and Veterinary Protozoology*. Publ. Churchill Livingstone, London.

Dubey, J. P. (1976). A review of *Sarcocystis* of domestic animals and of other coccidia of cats and dogs. J. Am. Vet. Med. Assoc., *169:* 1061-1078.

Dunn, A. M. (1978). *Veterinary Helminthology*. Publ. William Heinemann Medical Books Ltd., London.

Freeman, R. S., Stuart, P. F., Cullen, J. B., Ritchie, A. C., Mildon, A., Fernandes, B. J., and Bonin, R. (1976). Fatal human infection with mesocercariae of the trematode *Alaria americana*. Am. J. Trop. Med. Hyg., *25:* 803-807.

Georgi, J. R. (1974). *Parasitology for Veterinarians*. Publ. W. B. Saunders Company, Philadelphia.

Holmes, J. C., Carney, W. P., and Wood, C. E. (1970). Studies on sylvatic echinococcosis. III. Host occurrence and geographic distribution of *Echinococcus multilocularis* in the North Central United States. J. Parasitol., *56:* 1141-1150.

Jacobs, D. E., Pegg, E. J., and Stevenson, P. (1977). Helminths of British dogs: *Toxocara canis*— a veterinary perspective. J. Small Anim. Prac., *18:* 79-92.

Levine, N. D. (1968). *Nematode Parasites of Domestic Animals and Man*. Publ. Burgess Publishing Co., Minneapolis.

——————————(1973) *Protozoan Parasites of Domestic Animals and Man*. Publ. Burgess Publishing Co., Minneapolis.

Miller, T. A. (1971). Vaccination against the canine hookworm diseases. Adv. Parasitol., *9:* 153-184.

Nowell, I. (1978). *The Dog Crisis*. Publ. St. Martin's Press, Inc., New York.

Schantz, P. M., and Glickman, L. T. (1978). Toxocaral visceral larva migrans. New Eng. J. Med., *298*(8): 436-439.

Soulsby, E. J. L. (1968). *Helminths, Arthropods and Protozoa of Domesticated Animals (Monnig)*. Publ. Lea & Febiger, Philadelphia.

Teutsch, S. M., Juranek, D. D., Sulzer, A., Dubey, J. P., and Sikes, R. K. (1979). Epidemic toxoplasmosis associated with infected cats. New Eng. J. Med., *300*(13): 695-699.

Index